Music Therapy, and
Parent–Infant Bonding

Music Therapy and Parent–Infant Bonding

Edited by

Jane Edwards

OXFORD
UNIVERSITY PRESS

OXFORD

UNIVERSITY PRESS

Great Clarendon Street, Oxford OX2 6DP
United Kingdom

Oxford University Press is a department of the University of Oxford.
It furthers the University's objective of excellence in research, scholarship,
and education by publishing worldwide. Oxford is a registered trade mark of
Oxford University Press in the UK and in certain other countries

First published 2011
Reprinted 2012

British Library Cataloguing in Publication Data
Data available

Library of Congress Cataloging in Publication Data
Data available

ISBN 978-0-19-958051-4

Printed and bound by CPI Group (UK) Ltd, Croydon, CR0 4YY

Whilst every effort has been made to ensure that the contents of this work
are as complete, accurate and up-to-date as possible at the date of writing,
Oxford University Press is not able to give any guarantee or assurance that
such is the case. Readers are urged to take appropriately qualified medical
advise in all cases. The information in this work is intended to be useful to the
general reader, but should not be used as a means of self-diagnosis or for the
prescription of medication.

This book is dedicated to
Dorothy Scott

Acknowledgements

The authors would like to thank all of the families who permitted the use of their stories in this book. They would also like to thank their work places and colleagues for supporting their efforts and work. All client names have been changed in the interests of confidentiality. The editor would like to thank Professor William O'Connor for reviewing the neuroscience commentary, and also Oonagh MacMahon for her tireless assistance with the early proofreading. Thanks are due to the wonderful team at OUP who kept this project on track, especially Martin Baum and Charlotte Green.

Contents

Contributors

Vicky Abad is the Founding Director of *Sing & Grow* and is currently the Strategic Relations Consultant to Playgroup Queensland. She has extensive clinical and research experience in the field of parent–child interactions and vulnerable families. Vicky has published and presented on her work in national and international journals and currently lectures at the University of Queensland.

Donna Berthelsen is a Professor in the School of Early Childhood at the Queensland University of Technology. She is a developmental psychologist engaged in research that focuses on child outcomes in relation to family environments, early childhood education programmes, and early intervention programmes. Her research informs social and educational policy and practice.

Helen Bruderer is a qualified social worker currently working at Nambour General Hospital, Sunshine Coast, Queensland in the Women's and Paediatric Units as the Social Work Advanced Practitioner. Prior to this post she has predominately been involved in the areas of parenting for vulnerable families, child abuse, domestic violence and trauma.

Margareta Burrell is a music educator and music therapist who has specialized with children and their families for the past 30 years. She has worked at Thomas Coram Children's Centre since 2000 and is a member of the music therapy team at Coram, London. She is interested in the overlap between community music and music therapy.

Joanna Cunningham is a qualified music therapist. She worked at Familiscope in Ballyfermot, Dublin until March 2010. Joanna has developed an Early Intervention Arts Based Behavioural Support Programme called The SMARTS. This 14-session programme is funded from the Waterford Enterprise Board and is designed to be delivered in schools to small groups of Junior and Senior Infants who are struggling to adapt to primary school life.

Toni Day is the National Director of the *Sing & Grow* Project, Australia. She has worked as a music therapist for 15 years with a wide range of clinical populations, including with women and young people who have experienced trauma. She has completed her Masters degree on the experience of song writing as an intervention within a parenting programme for women who have experienced childhood abuse and has published on this work.

Louise Docherty is a registered music therapist currently working at The Royal Children's Hospital Melbourne with paediatric oncology patients. She has an interest in community and is currently undertaking PhD study that is exploring process evaluation in music therapy and community cultural development.

Tiffany Drake is the former Head of Coram's Music Therapy Service in London, UK. She completed an MPhil documenting her research into the efficacy of community-based music therapy and outcomes for children. She is currently pursuing her interest in attachment and infant communication closer to home as a mother to a toddler and baby twins.

Jane Edwards is the Director of the Music & Health Research Group at the University of Limerick where she heads the MA in Music Therapy training. She was formerly the course director for the music therapy programme at the University of Queensland. She is the inaugural President of the International Association for Music & Medicine.

Brigid Jordan is the Associate Professor of Paediatric Social Work (Infant and Family) at the Royal Children's Hospital, Melbourne and the Department of Paediatrics, The University of Melbourne. She also heads the Social and Mental Health Aspects of Serious Illness Research Group at the Murdoch Children's Research Institute.

Karen Kelly is a qualified music therapist and was previously employed at the Bluebox Creative Learning Centre in Limerick. She has experience of music therapy service provision in child and family work and mental health. She is currently working as a music therapist at the Milford Care Centre in Limerick, Ireland.

Alison Ledger is a qualified music therapist who has worked with children and families in a number of health and education settings. Since carrying out the work reported in her chapter she has completed her doctoral studies at the University of Limerick on the topic of music therapy service development.

Alison Levinge has a lifelong interest in early attachment issues. She began her career as a music therapist working with the internationally known Consultant Paediatrician Hugh Jolly at Charing Cross Child Development Centre, London. Alison pioneered the first Arts therapy training in Wales which she led for 11 years. Alison chaired the Bristol Psychotherapy Association for 12 years and continues to carry out her practice with children who have been bereaved.

Joanne V. Loewy is the Director of the Louis Armstrong Center for Music and Medicine at Beth Israel Medical Center in New York City. She is the co-Editor-in-Chief of the international peer reviewed journal *Music and Medicine*.

Jan M. Nicholson is the incoming Director of Research at the Parenting Research Centre in Melbourne, Principal Research Fellow at the Murdoch Children's Research Institute and Adjunct Associate Professor at the Centre for Learning Innovation, Queensland University of Technology. She has a background in child and family psychology with postdoctoral training in public health. Her research examines the influence of contemporary family, social and organizational environments on children's healthy development, with a particular focus on vulnerable families.

Clare O'Callaghan is a qualified music therapist and social worker. She works as a music therapist at Peter MacCallum Cancer Centre and Caritas Christi Hospice, St Vincent's Hospital, in Melbourne, Australia, and is widely published in practice-based research.

Amelia Oldfield has over 30 years' experience as a music therapist. She has been working with families for the past 22 years at a Child Development Centre and at a Unit for Child and Family Psychiatry. She is currently seeking to establish a new integrated service in the NHS for families and young children with developmental problems to provide emotional support for the families around the time of diagnosis.

Helen Shoemark has worked as a music therapist for more than 30 years, and has been at The Royal Children's Hospital Melbourne since 1995, where she is the senior therapist for neonates and infants. As a researcher in the Murdoch Children's Research Institute, Helen's research focuses on inter-personal interventions with infants and families and the application of music and music therapy for high risk newborn infants. She is currently an Adjunct Professor with the School of Music, University of Queensland.

Kate E. Williams was the Deputy National Director of *Sing & Grow* from 2005 to 2007 and is currently the Research & Policy Manager for Playgroup Queensland. She has recently completed a research Masters project which examined the effectiveness of group music therapy for parents who have a young child with a disability. Kate is currently undertaking research in to the ways infant temperament and self-regulation skills interact with parenting and parent mental health to produce social and emotional outcomes for young children.

Abbreviations

ACS	Association for Child Services
CSA	childhood sexual abuse
NAS	neonatal abstinence syndrome
NICU	neonatal intensive care unit
NIDCP	Newborn Individualized Developmental Care and Assessment Program
NNU	neonatal unit
NOS	neonatal opium solution
PTSS	post-traumatic stress symptoms
RCH	The Royal Children's Hospital Melbourne
RDS	respiratory distress syndrome

Introduction

Jane Edwards

From the first beat of your heart in utero you become a rhythmic being. From the first cry on entering the world you discover the undulations of melody, and from the first playful vocal interactions with a caregiver your capacity for relating begins its lifelong harmony.

We have all seen and heard how an adult interacting with a baby will raise their vocal pitch, repeat words, elongate vowels, and start a sing-song dialogue with the baby using animated facial expressions. It is a delight to watch the infant respond to these playful cues for interaction; first by attending and then increasingly by smiling, imitating and engaging in a call and response encounter. The baby is highly skilled in these kinds of interactions, and increasingly it has been demonstrated that these music-like interactions between a caregiver and infant strengthen and promote the necessary developmental progress of the infant and young child.

This book presents the ways in which music therapists have come to understand their unique role in promoting healthy relating between the infant and their primary caregiver in order to attain successful attachment. An established body of international research indicates that these experiences of communication and relating in the early years of life are crucial to successful developmental outcomes in later childhood through to adulthood.

Aims and purpose of the book

As the first book in the music therapy literature to focus primarily on the ways professionals in this field use their skills for the promotion of attachment between vulnerable caregivers and infants, this book complements recent texts that have shown the developing theoretical and applied aspects of music in infancy, and in music therapy with families (Malloch and Trevarthen 2008;

Oldfield and Flower 2008). This text aims to fill a much needed gap to provide further support for teaching, practice and ongoing evaluation of parent–infant bonding in music therapy; ultimately presenting a greater awareness of the need for funded research that can inform policy and practice.

Contemporary music therapy practices are presented in each chapter along with engaging descriptions of the ways in which vulnerability in attachment and bonding between a parent and their infant are addressed, and their capacities strengthened. Music therapy practices in four countries, Australia, Ireland, the UK, and the USA, are presented, providing an overview of active new approaches within established models by a range of authors, many of whom are well recognized as international experts in this field. Current theoretical models used to develop and inform effective music therapy practices in a range of contexts are also outlined. The clinical material complements other infant mental health publications and work internationally in clinical psychology, psychiatry, child development, and education.

For students of music therapy, the book can offer an overview of contemporary practitioners approach to work with vulnerable parents and infants. For music therapy practitioners, it is hoped that further understanding of the work is elaborated and appreciated. In the wider context of parent–infant research and practice it is hoped this text will offer an opportunity to discover common ground and explore new possibilities for research and practice together.

Overview of the structure

The book comprises three sections: (i) music therapy research and practice to ameliorate vulnerability in infancy; (ii) descriptions of successful group music therapy programmes; and (iii) music therapy work with parents and infants in medical settings. Each chapter can be read without reference to the rest of the book, and each of the three sections can stand alone for use in referencing specialist aspects of the book. However, music therapy students, practitioners and researchers are encouraged to read as much of the book as possible since it is the first overview text providing a unique insight into the parameters of this developing approach. It is hoped that the book will spark greater interest in the capacity of music therapy professionals to provide expert therapy interventions at a most crucial time of development.

Background to the text

Personally, this book reflects a long time passion about the contribution of music therapy to the work of parent–infant bonding. My first music therapy student placement in a pre-school for children with vision impairment and multiple handicap brought parents and their infants together in sessions. During my clinical training placement in Cambridge in the late 1980s I had the opportunity to observe weekly sessions in the Addenbrooke's Child Development Unit with Dr Amelia Oldfield. Parents and infants were seen together for assessment and therapy. On return to Australia I studied a family theory module in the social work department at Melbourne University with Professor Dorothy Scott. My research and clinical work at the Royal Children's Hospital in Brisbane from 1993 to 2000 was especially informed from this theoretical training.

Early on in my work with children and their families at the Royal Children's Hospital I remember presenting a case report at a seminar and during the question time a colleague asked me 'Don't you find that the families get in the way?' I then realized there was still more work to be done in helping students and practitioners in music therapy, and more widely, to be better equipped to realize and promote the benefits of family centred practice.

In her visit to Brisbane in 2000 Dr Joanne Loewy gave an expert engaging presentation about the parent–infant groups that she led. Some months later when opening the newspaper on a Sunday morning I noticed a call for expressions of interest in applying for federal funding to develop new programmes to support vulnerable parents and their young children. Along with my music therapy colleague at the University of Queensland, Brandy Walker, and in association with Playgroups Queensland, I wrote a funding proposal for the parent–infant music therapy service *Sing & Grow* which is now a national programme in Australia; Vicky Abad served as the inaugural director. Since moving permanently to Ireland I have had the opportunity to be involved in the development of a number of further parent–infant projects some of which appear in the following chapters.

The families described in this book are experiencing life challenges for which their available resources overwhelm their ability to cope. The work of music therapists to support and ameliorate these challenges in order to promote a healthy bond between parent and infant is richly described and the successful outcomes celebrated.

References

Malloch, S., and Trevarthen, C. (2008). Musicality: communicating the vitality and interest of life. In S. Malloch, and C. Trevarthen (eds) *Communicative Musicality: Exploring the Basis for Human Companionship*, pp. 1–11. (Oxford: Oxford University Press)

Oldfield, A., and Flower, C. (2008). *Music Therapy with Children and their Families*. (London: Jessica Kingsley)

Chapter 1

Music therapy and parent–infant bonding

Jane Edwards

Building the bonds of love in a secure relationship in the early years is considered essential to making a good start in life. Part of the repertory of interaction involves easily identified music elements. This predisposes the music therapist to having a strong basis on which to support therapeutic interventions that promote secure bonding between vulnerable infants and their caregivers. By providing a musical container, or skin, in which both the parent and infant can be held, music therapy can offer the dyad a chance to safely encounter and explore one another anew. Music therapists have rich resources for supporting this capacity sensitively and joyfully with their clients.

This chapter presents some of the theoretical formations and research that supports the work of qualified music therapists in promoting healthy and secure attachment between parents and infants where disruption to a secure relational bond has occurred, or is vulnerable in some way. Characteristics of the innate musicality of the very young infant are considered, and the mutual regulation potentials of music making between caregivers and their developing infants is discussed. For the purposes of this chapter, and indeed this book, the definition of infant used is the broadest possible; from birth until 3 years and 11 months of age.

In a healthy relationship the caregiver '. . . affords emotional access to the child and responds appropriately and promptly to his or her positive and negative states.' (Schore 2001 p. 205). This supports the adaptation of the infant towards internal regulation functions which relate to 'the regulation of arousal, the maintenance of alertness, the capacity to dampen arousal in the face of over-stimulation, the capacity to inhibit behavioral expression, and the capacity to develop predictable behavioral cycles.' (Beebe and Lachmann 1998 p. 485). This interpersonal and intrapsychic regulation of the parent–infant dyad is considered interactive; 'Interactive regulation flows in both directions, on a moment-to-moment basis, so that each experiences influencing, as well as being influenced by, the other's behavior.' (Beebe and Lachmann 1998 p. 500). The caregiver–infant system is considered a developing dyadic or triadic structure (Corboz-Warnery et al. 1993; Stern 2000) with one or both parents or other caregivers playing an essential role in the formation of a secure base in interaction with the infant. The infant's need for external support is evident, leading Winnicott to deduce that 'there is no such thing as a baby' (Winnicott 1952 p. 99). That is, a baby depends for its survival on being part of a care system involving one or more adults who have responsibility for providing security, support, and nurture. As Ham and Tronick (2009) have described, infants '. . . require regulatory input from others to sustain even basic homeostatic and physiological processes such as body temperature, sleep cycles digestion and motor stability' (p. 621). The newborn is highly capable of communicating needs such as hunger and fatigue, and the responsive caregiver supports these needs.

As Schore has elegantly stated, 'Development may be conceptualized as the transformation of external into internal regulation' (Schore 2001 p. 205). Through the early years the infant depends on external support to develop the capacity for managing their internal state. Interpersonal and intrapsychic regulation are crucial to a healthy start to life, and these processes are interdependent (Beebe and Lachmann 1998).

Promoting the use of music as a means to enjoy and explore parent–infant relations is not new. However, the impact of music therapy interventions on the development of the bonds of attachment is increasingly of interest within the music therapy community of practitioners working with vulnerable parents and infants, especially in the early intervention setting (Jonsdottir 2002; Edwards et al. 2007; Nicholson et al. 2008).

Music therapy

Many descriptions of the use of music in health and healing contexts have appeared in the historical record prior to the formalization of the field now known as music therapy (Gouk 2000; Edwards 2007). The current established professionalization of music therapy primarily developed in the twentieth century as a post-war phenomenon. 'Musical therapy' was enthusiastically championed by musicians and music teachers to support the needs of the large numbers of returned servicemen from the two World Wars (Edwards 2007; Sullivan 2007).

This led to calls from qualified healthcare professionals for appropriate and specialized training to be provided in order to practice music therapy. The resultant development of university-based courses around the world from the mid 1940s can be traced to the recognition that a range of psychosocial care needs were able to be addressed through interactions and opportunities observed and recorded in the music sessions in which these returned soldiers participated (Edwards 2007).

The field of music therapy has subsequently benefited from theoretical perspectives provided from psychoanalysis (Streeter 1999), humanistic psychology (Noone 2008), and therapeutic approaches to the treatment of psychological distress (Edwards and Kennelly 2011). Providing a therapeutic relationship with a qualified practitioner where co-created music making is the basis of interaction has been shown to provide therapeutic benefits for people receiving care in many medical, community, and education settings. Research studies and reviews have shown that music therapy is effective for many client groups including people who have mental disorders (Edwards 2006), children who have autism (Gold et al. 2006), pain management for burn patients (Tan 2010), and for people who have dementia (Raglio et al. 2008).

Parent–infant work in music therapy has gradually developed as a professional interest with recognized leaders (Abad and Williams 2007; Oldfield and Flower 2008; Shoemark and Dearn 2008), and specialist conferences. As in other related therapy practices, music therapists began to see the benefits and relevance of the inclusion of family members in work with children, and expanded their practice to treat dyads (Oldfield 1995; Trolldalen 1997). Music therapy programmes for the support of attachment behaviours between vulnerable parents and their infants have been founded, notably the Australian programme *Sing & Grow* (Abad and Edwards 2004; Abad and Williams 2005, 2007).

In the context of parent–infant work, music therapy can be described as a process of developing a relationship with a caregiver/dyad in order to support, develop, and extend their skills in using musical and music-like interactions including vocal improvisation, chants, lullabies, songs, and rhymes, to promote and enhance the sensitivity and mutual co-regulation between infant and caregiver, in order to create the optimal environment for secure attachment to be fostered. Music therapy for parent–infant bonding is practised in groups, and in dyad- or triad-based parent–infant sessions.

In the Australian programme *Sing & Grow* music therapy is offered through short-term weekly sessions for groups of up to 10 families (Abad and Williams 2007). The purpose of music therapy is to 'strengthen parent-child relationships through increasing developmentally conducive interactions, by assisting parents to bond with their children, and by extending the repertory of parenting skills in relating to their child through interactive play' (Abad and Williams 2007 p. 52).

The musically primed infant

Extensive research studies have identified distinctive and surprising aspects of early musical capacity in the human infant. It is well established that the newborn infant can distinguish elements of rhythm, pitch, and melody (Papoušek 1996). As they develop, infants use this knowledge to learn about the world around them, and to acquire language (Vosoughi et al. 2010).

Newborn cries recorded within five days of birth showed that German and French infants differed in the contour of their cries (Mampe et al. 2009). The French babies produced cries with a predominantly rising contour, and the German babies showed a falling contour in their crying. These findings suggest that infants are influenced by the rise and fall in the tonality of the language they hear spoken while in the hearing phase of their development *in utero* (Mampe et al. 2009).

Infants' early cry stabilizes at a pitch that is relatively constant with individual infants showing only a semitone variation by 3 months of age (Wermke et al. 2002). These findings have indicated that for the human infant 'linguistic and musical channels are likely to be equally accessible and not discrete' (Cross 2009). This suggests that infants may not be discriminating between music and speech but instead are drawn to the types of vocal interplay that they experience as more meaningful and recognizable.

There is a substantial body of evidence to show that infants prefer music to speech. They especially show preference for their own mother's singing rather than her speaking (Nakata and Trehub 2004), and prefer this singing when it has infant-directed features (Trainor 1996).

In a study of fathers singing, infants did not show a greater preference for either audiovisual recordings of their father's singing that was infant-directed, or for songs recorded without the infant present (O'Neill et al. 2001). In the same study a comparison of infants who watched a recording of their father's singing and their mother's singing, indicated that infants paid greater visual attention to fathers (O'Neill et al. 2001). Informal observation led the researchers to propose that this may have been due to some performance elements of the father's singing described as 'vigorous' and 'exuberant' with elements of self-consciousness that were not perceived in the mother's performance (O'Neill et al. 2001 p. 422).

Other examinations of musical preference in infancy have shown further discrimination abilities. In tests of 6- and 7-month-old infants using head turning as a measure of preference it was demonstrated that unfamiliar lullabies were preferred when sung at a lower pitch and unfamiliar playsongs were preferred when sung at a higher pitch (Tsang and Conrad 2010). Previous research showed infants preferred lower pitched renditions of unfamiliar lullabies

(Volkova et al. 2006). Even at the age of 2 months infants have been shown to remember a short melody and then be able to distinguish between the familiar melody and a novel melodic phrase (Plantinga and Trainor 2009).

The infant's musical capacities develop alongside all of their rapidly progressing motor, language, and social developmental changes in the early years. Musical skill acquisition has a regular developmental sequence (Hargreaves 1982; Briggs 1991). Briggs used an extensive literature base of studies of music in the early years to propose a phased model charting this development in the four areas of capacity: (1) auditory; (2) vocal/tonal; (3) rhythmic; and (4) cognitive. Infants first use their abilities in listening and vocalizing during the 'reflex phase' from birth to 9 months. They then develop skills in being able to copy musical phrases and learn snatches of songs during the 'intention phase' until around 18 months. The next 18 months of the 'control phase' shows rapid development of the ability to control musical elements, and in the final 'integration phase' they are able to learn a music instrument, and rapidly learn songs, rhymes, rhythms, and chants (Briggs 1991).

As with language abilities, perception and reception develop first and then the ability to perform musical tasks including singing and the use of instruments (for a review see Miyamoto 2007). Loewy (1995) elaborated the musical stages of speech development in a study of the pre-verbal skills in infancy and the relationship of these to music therapy work with clients who do not speak. As hearing, vocalizations, and the musical perceptual system is well developed in infancy, it is common sense to consider the ways in which musical play can offer a means to engage and communicate with vulnerable infants.

The musical parent

Since the infant has the neurological and auditory maturity to discriminate pitch and to increasingly recognize the emotional intention of vocal timbre (Bergeson and Trehub 1999), it is understandable that caregivers worldwide soon realize that the infant will best attend and respond to requests for playful interactions when offered through stereotypical 'sing-song' vocalizations. This particular way of singing and speaking when interacting with infants in order to capture their attention and promote reciprocity (Bergeson and Trehub 1999; Bryant and Barrett 2007) is known as 'infant-directed'[1] in that it is distinct from the way adults use their voice in interaction with older children and with each other (Trehub et al. 1993). The way that the infant responds to this playing easily promotes feelings of loving intimacy for the caregiver which is vital to bonding (Gerhardt 2004). For example, this 'emotional musicality' or

---

[1] Previously termed 'motherese' or 'baby talk'.

singing quality was not present in an acoustic analysis of the vocalizing of a depressed mother as compared with a mother with no mood disturbance (Robb 1999), and a review of studies of interactions between parents and infants from 3 to 6 months of age showed that depressed mothers use less infant-directed speech, and have difficulties with the synchrony of their timing in vocal interplay with their babies (Field 2010).

Prosody is the rise and fall of pitch in speaking that is similar to the pitch changes in a melody. Adults use distinctive pitches and exaggerated prosodic contours in producing infant-directed speech. Infant-directed singing similarly includes features such as 'final phrase syllable lengthening' (Trainor 1996 p. 89), placing emphasis on certain words, and using a 'loving tone of voice' (p. 90), that is probably a function of smiling while singing (Trainor 1996). This type of singing is used by children as young as 3 years of age when singing to younger siblings (Trehub et al. 1994).

It has been demonstrated that individual mothers create distinct 'signature tunes' (Bergeson and Trehub 2007) by using the same pitch in the rise and fall of their utterances to their infants. Caregivers 'across cultures use broadly similar pitch contours to express their arousing, soothing, and disapproving intentions . . .' (Bergeson and Trehub 2007 p. 648). It is proposed that this pitch stability creates a way for the infant to recognize the mother's voice and this recognition serves to 'enhance reciprocal emotional ties' (Bergeson and Trehub 2007 p. 649).

Mothers singing songs to their 4- to 7-month-old infants recorded 1 week apart were shown to produce the exact pitch and rhythm in both renditions (Bergeson and Trehub 2007). Adult capacities for pitch perception, recognition, and recall have been shown to be stable even in people who have not developed absolute pitch[2] and do not have musical training (Schellenberg and Trehub 2003; Levitin and Rogers 2005) suggesting that this ability is retained and continues to be used as a perceptual skill beyond infancy.

Many parents also learn that a lullaby can be used to aid relaxation, soothe distress, and invite sleep (Trehub and Trainor 1998). However, the lullaby is rarely used as an exclusive soother in promoting sleep. For example, in a study of the experiences of using lullabies for 18 first time mothers, MacKinlay and Baker (2005) found that 'Patting, stroking, rocking, bouncing, or walking around the room while singing to babies were common techniques . . .' (MacKinlay and Baker 2005 p. 88). Music and movement are allies when searching for ways to soothe and comfort a tired infant.

Malloch and Trevarthen (2008) have linked this parent–infant 'musicality' metaphorically to movement citing evidence to support their view that we

---

[2] Absolute pitch is the ability to attach a letter name to a note on hearing the note played.

'live, think, imagine and remember in movement' (Malloch and Trevarthen 2008 p. 1). In music therapy work with mothers and their infants it has been noted that the function of 'recognition' between parent and infant requires the presence of sound, gesture and movement (Trolldalen 1997); 'That is, timing, . . . dynamics, . . . and narrativity' (Trolldalen 1997 p. 26). Additionally Papoušek has noted that these musical interactions between parents and their infants are usually multimodal, not only involving auditory-based melodic and vocal interplay but also having rhythmic, physical movement, and visual aspects (Papoušek 1996). So while this chapter explores the capacities of musical interaction and music-like interactions in parent–infant bonding, it is recognized that non-verbal and tactile aspects of this interaction are present for the parent and infant when learning each other's 'rhythmic structure' (Schore 2009).

Musical relating in parent–infant communication

Malloch and Trevarthen (2008) described four decades of mainly observational research about playful communicative interactions between mothers and infants. They noted how interactions were observed by many researchers to be highly ritualized, leading to descriptions of these interactions as 'musical' or 'dance like' (Malloch and Trevarthen 2008 p. 1). For example Papoušek noted how in transcribing infant-directed speech into pitch classes she was tempted to also record the musical 'connotations' of these interactions 'such as crescendo/diminuendo, rallentando/accelerando, legato/staccato, dolce, or agitato' (Papoušek 1996 p. 94). As the music therapist Mercédès Pavlicevic has noted, parents and infants create highly expressive interactions where both partners 'negotiate and share a flexible musical pulse between them, constantly adapting their tempi, intensity, motion, shape and contour of their sounds, movements and gestures in order to "fit" with the communicating partner' (Pavlicevic 2000 p. 274)

As the infant does not have a shared understanding of words, considering these vocally playful interactions between parents and pre-verbal infants to have musical characteristics and qualities adds a useful dimension in examining the functions and benefits of these exchanges. Papoušek has proposed that adults use of these melodic contours in infant-directed speech is a 'communicative code' (Papoušek 1996 p. 96). This 'communicative musicality' (Malloch 1999) affords the infant and caregiver a way to express and exchange information about emotional states; fundamental to strengthening the bonds of love.

Stern has explained that the success of the adult's interaction with the infant is generally dependent on three aspects; 'the extent of their repertoire of infant-elicited social behaviours; the manner of performance of these behaviours (richness, variety, and fullness of displays); and the subtlety of timing of these behaviours so they are most effective' (Stern 1977 p. 41). This playful interaction has further been noted to have the temporal features of 'signalling, synchrony, and attunement' (Ham and Tronick 2009 p. 620). Since all musical performance requires attention to timing, pitch and synchrony, musical elements can easily be heard in the playful interactions between caregivers and infants.

Trehub has observed that in relation to caregiver and infant music making 'Music is not communicative in the sense of sharing information. Instead, it is concerned with sharing feelings and experiences and the regulation of social behaviour' (Trehub 2003 p. 672). This capacity of musical exchanges such as singing nursery songs or lullabies to convey feeling states offers a means to experience mutually satisfying and meaningful interactions, and is therefore highly relevant to the practice of music therapy in parent–infant work. Additionally, the musical qualities of vocal interplay between parents and pre-verbal infants has a resonance with the type of improvised music created in music therapy with patients of all ages (Pavlicevic 2000).

Through observing minute by minute interactions between parents and infants during their long research careers Colwyn Trevarthen (2001a, 2001b) and Daniel Stern (2000) have found that 'communication with an infant is, from the beginning, intersubjective and emotional, valuable to both infant and adult in itself as an interpersonal exchange of feelings and state of animation, no matter what the language content' (Trevarthen 2001a p. 103). Influenced by her doctoral studies with Daniel Stern, Beatrice Beebe also pursued an extensive research career making links between early face to face parent–infant interactions and the capacities for psychoanalytic therapy to offer support and change to vulnerable adults (Beebe and Lachmann 1998).

Stephen Malloch is a trained musician who worked with Colwyn Trevarthen as a postdoctoral researcher in the 1990s. While watching and listening to recordings of interactions between mothers and their infants he was struck by the musical aspects of these co-created events leading him to suggest that '. . . a mother and her infant can jointly create a musical piece–both are musical partners within their communication space' (Malloch 1999 p. 47). Malloch and Trevarthen concluded that 'these "musical" narratives allow adult and infant, and adult and adult to share a sense of sympathy and situated meaning in a shared sense of passing time' (Malloch and Trevarthen 2008 p. 4).

Dissanayake also noted the musicality of these communicative encounters. She proposed that this playful interaction is 'proto-musical' and is a foundation source for the universals of human musical behaviour (Dissanayake 2008). In her view, the proto-musical features of 'formalization, repetition, exaggeration, dynamic variation, and manipulation of expectation' (p. 176) contribute to emotional bonding because they impact on the infants 'visual, vocal, and kinesic signals that enable their emotional bond with their mother' (Dissanayake 2008 p. 176).

The use of these musical elements to co-create mutually satisfying encounters between parents and their offspring is increasingly understood to contribute to healthy and optimal growth through the early years; and these positive interactions in turn create a strong foundation for future capacities for intimacy and positive relating, with these positive early relations influencing later mental health (Maselko et al. 2010).

Parent–infant bonding

It might seem unnecessary in a contemporary presentation of this topic to search for evidence that a supportive, secure, and intimate relationship with a primary caregiver is an essential start to healthy progression through life. However, many theorists in the middle of the twentieth century devoted their working lives to proving the essential role of attachment in infancy. A summary of the necessity for attachment can found in the British psychiatrist John Bowlby's report to the World Health Organization (Bowlby 1951). 'The infant and young child should experience a warm, intimate, and continuous relationship with his mother (or permanent mother substitute) in which both find satisfaction and enjoyment' (Bowlby 1951 p. 13). Mary Ainsworth (Ainsworth et al. 1978) and James Robertson (Bowlby and Robertson 1952; Robertson 1953) worked with John Bowlby to gather evidence that maternal deprivation caused significant stress for infants and young children with lifelong consequences. Although it took decades to achieve, their research findings changed hospital practices to allow parents visiting rights (van der Horst and van der Veer 2010), and became influential in how the needs of vulnerable children were perceived (Bretherton 1992).

Throughout the last century a series of influential figures gave further credence to the necessity for a secure parent–infant base to support the development of lifelong capacities for psychological stability and the capacity to form intimate relationships successfully with others (Winnicott 1965; Beebe and Lachmann 1998; Stern 2000; Trevarthen 2001a). It has become increasingly evident that attachment behaviours have specific purposes and require sensitivity and responsiveness on the part of the caregiver. The figure of the mother or other primary carer must behave in what Winnicott has described as a 'good enough' way to contain the infant's anxieties and fears of: (1) going to pieces: (2) falling for ever; (3) having no relationship to the body; (4) having no orientation; and (5) complete isolation because there is no way to communicate (Winnicott 1965 p. 58)

The development of the ability to relate and communicate has been described as a series of building blocks or developmental phases of intrapsychic and interpersonal capacity that he described as having various 'domains' that include the 'Emergent self' from birth until 2 months, 'Core self' from 2 to 6 months, the 'Subjective self' that emerges in the period from 7 to 15 months, the 'Verbal self' at 15–18 months, and then the 'Narrative self' at around 3–3.5 years (Stern 2000 p. xxv).

The expectation of the infant that emotionally sensitive interplay will be available to them is supported by experiments where mothers were instructed to play with their 1-year-old infants and then present a blank and motionless face for some minutes while still staring at their infant (Ham and Tronick 2009). The resultant behavioural response from the infant can include fussing, crying and general perturbation until the mother re-engages again. The results from measures of skin conductance and respiratory sinus arrhythmia showed that at re-engagement the mother first calmed herself, and then calmed her baby. This finding provides support for the hypothesis that mutual co-regulation supports the infant's emotional equilibrium (Ham and Tronick 2009).[3]

When the ability to seek or maintain this communication is absent or impaired in the relationship urgent support and help is needed. A qualified music therapist can work in gentle non-intrusive ways to help parents and their infants discover and strengthen their capacity for relating through the musical play that is part of the usual repertory of parent–infant interactions.

Parent–infant music therapy

It is difficult to trace the exact starting point for music therapists' interest in providing supportive parent–infant interventions to vulnerable infants and their carers. Abad and Edwards (2004) reported the start up of the *Sing & Grow* programme in Australia and proposed that 'the use of music therapy to assist parents to extend their repertory of successful and nurturing parental behaviours in interaction with their young children' was 'relatively new' (Abad and Edwards 2004 p. 14), and 'under reported and researched' (p. 5). Oldfield and Bunce (2001) had also described that music therapy work with mothers and young children was unusual. Family-centred music therapy had been provided in a playgroup programme with early intervention goals some years earlier in Australia (Shoemark 1996).

---

3 When this study was presented at a NICU Summit at Beth Israel Hospital New York (Ham 2010) footage was presented of a dyad where the infant turned the still face part of the experiment into a game, becoming highly vocally humorous and eventually repeatedly 'breaking' his mother's motionless face resulting in both of them, and indeed the summit delegates, collapsing into helpless laughter.

Music therapists have reported work with families in a range of contexts. The medical settings of the Neonatal Intensive Care Unit, and work in burns and oncology have particularly highlighted the need for an understanding of the role of the family as a central resource as well as the focus for music therapy interventions (Edwards 1998; Daveson and Kennelly 2000; Shoemark and Dearn 2008; Stewart 2009).

Many music therapists have noted the connections between the creation of music in the client–therapist relationship in music therapy and early mother–infant interactions (Hughes 1995; Pavlicevic 2000). Therefore, the adult's experience in infancy of the capacity to develop a creative vocal dialogue is considered by some to be reflected later in the relationship evolving in the musical interactions in music therapy. Diane Austin, for example, has described her music therapy approach as 'vocal psychotherapy' (Austin 2008). She has suggested that certain types of vocal techniques in the early stages of therapy work with adults are often similar to parent–infant vocalizations, giving the patient the opportunity to experience 'an emotionally present, attuned mother' (Austin 2008 p. 149).

A music therapy pilot project sought to determine the effects of structured group music involvement with children between the age of 12 and 24 months and their parents (Standley et al. 2009). Findings showed that children in the music group benefited in cognitive and musical development compared with matched controls. This study included parents and so is of interest to this chapter. However, the focus of the study is on infants' developmental skills rather than parent–infant interactions. In comparison, Abad and Williams (2007) reported the benefits of supporting parents in group music therapy programmes to engage musically with their young children to promote attachment. A report of a music therapy group programme with self-referred 'well' families reported benefits with offering social support and additional ways to deal with parental challenges (Mackenzie and Hamlet 2005). Other music therapy programmes with mothers and their infants have shown benefits in the quality of interaction observed, and self reported satisfaction with participation in the sessions (Oldfield and Bunce 2001; Oldfield et al. 2003). Observations in music therapy sessions with mothers and their infants from the asylum seeker community in Limerick, Ireland showed that interactions and interpersonal engagement improved for these vulnerable, 'preoccupied' mothers and their children (Edwards et al. 2007).

Additionally, Bargiel (2004) has made a number of recommendations about the development of early intervention music therapy programmes to support parents and their infants. Specifically she proposed that the first interaction be the therapist and dyad, with a group programme only commencing after twice weekly sessions for 10 weeks and a follow-up assessment (Bargiel 2004).

The first study to evaluate a short-term early intervention music therapy parent–infant programme using validated measures found that for 358 parents and infants, a number of significant benefits impacted the parent and child in a range of areas including education in the home and parental mental health (Nicholson et al. 2008).

Conclusion

Building the bonds of love in a secure relationship in the early years is considered essential to making a good start in life. Part of the repertory of interaction in a loving parent–infant relationship involves easily identified music elements. This predisposes the music therapist to having a strong basis on which to support therapeutic interventions that promote secure bonding between vulnerable infants and their caregivers.

Parent–infant interactions do not necessarily have musical intention but recognition of the musical features of this interplay provokes further reflection about music therapy dynamics. The process of musical improvisation in music therapy sessions reveals much about the communicative relationship available between the client and therapist (Pavlicevic 2000). The music created can be considered a 'by-product' rather than being the intended outcomes of the work of building the relationship between the therapist and client (John 1992). The music therapist works with the client to evoke musical narratives of his or her emotional and interpersonal life experiences (Austin 2008). The music that is created is less relevant as a cultural symbol than a deeply affective emotional communication channel. For a child or adult with a disability that has prevented their development of language as a means of communication, this interaction offers a 'lifeline to human sociality' (Malloch and Trevarthen 2008 p. 6). For adults seeking support for psychological distress, it is possible that in the incoherence they experience in trying to make meaning from what they feel, this musical interaction can offer a supportive holding place for the incomprehensible of the feeling world until it is ready, like the infant's eventual development of words, to become the story that can be told.

By providing a musical container, or skin, in which both the parent and infant can be held, music therapy can offer the dyad a chance to safely encounter and explore one another anew. Music therapists have rich resources for supporting this capacity sensitively and joyfully with their clients. Further research and development work is needed in order to understand how to optimize and promote this work more widely, especially with the inclusion of potential co-collaborators from related disciplines.

Further distinctions between and a deeper understanding of theoretical approaches will help in providing specific training and supervision support for

practitioners. For example, distinctions and the overlap between music therapy as a preventive approach or as a treatment approach are not always clear.
The role of the therapeutic relationship between the therapist and the dyad and
how this is established, fostered, and maintained in a music therapy context,
including in group programmes, could be further elaborated. Measurement
and evaluation of outcomes has received some attention (Nicholson et al.
2008; Standley et al. 2009). However, standardized evaluation tools for routine
use in music therapy parent–infant programmes could be usefully developed.

Since it is possible that anyone can sing with a baby it is sometimes challenging
to claim expertise in musical interactions, and to promote the benefits of and
need for a particular music therapy perspective. Increasingly musicians and
musical organizations promote a range of add-on benefits for music in society
and daily life in order to justify access to public funding (Edwards 2010).
Negotiating our shared interests while claiming a distinct specialist role without
marginalizing or becoming marginsalized can be challenging. As we add our voices
to the community of therapy practitioners who care for and offer support to
vulnerable caregivers and their infants, it is hoped that the points of connection
will be stronger than any moments of divergence, and that the developing
nature of this work can be given due credence and opportunity.

References

Abad, V., and Edwards, J. (2004). Strengthening families: A role for music therapy in
contributing to family centred care. *Australian Journal of Music Therapy*, 15, 3–16.

Abad, V., and Williams, K. (2005). Early intervention music therapy for adolescent mothers
and their hildren. *British Journal of Music Therapy*, 19, 31–38.

Abad, V., and Williams, K. (2007). Early intervention music therapy: reporting on a 3-year
project to address needs with at-risk families. *Music Therapy Perspectives*, 25, 52–58.

Ainsworth, M., Blehar, M., Waters, E., and Wall, S. (1978). *Patterns of Attachment: a
Psychological Study of the Strange Situation*. (Hillsdale, NJ: Erlbaum)

Austin, D. (2008). *The Theory and Practice of Vocal Psychotherapy: Songs of the Self*.
(London: Jessica Kingsley)

Bargiel, M. (2004). Lullabies and play songs: theoretical considerations for an early attachment
music therapy intervention through parental singing for developmentally at-risk infants.
Voices: a World Forum for Discussion, 4 np. Available at https://normt.uib.no/index.
php/voices/article/viewArticle/149/125. Accessed January 2011.

Beebe, B., and Lachmann, F. (1998). Co-constructing inner and relational processes: Self and
mutual regulation in infant research and adult treatment. *Psychoanalytic Psychology*, 15,
480–516.

Bergeson, T., and Trehub, S.E. (1999). Mothers' singing to infants and preschool children.
Infant Behavior and Development, 22, 51–64.

Bergeson, T.R., and Trehub, S.E. (2007). Signature tunes in mothers' speech to infants.
Infant Behavior and Development, 30, 648–654.

Bowlby, J. (1951). Maternal care and mental health. *Bulletin of the World Health Organization*, 3, 353–534.

Bowlby, J., and Robertson, J. (1952). A two-year-old goes to hospital. *Proceedings of the Royal Society for Medicine*, 46, 425–427.

Bretherton, I. (1992). The origins of attachment theory: John Bowlby and Mary Ainsworth. *Developmental Psychology*, 28, 759–775.

Briggs, C. (1991). A model for understanding musical development. *Music Therapy*, 10, 1–21.

Bryant, G., and Barrett, C. (2007). Recognizing intentions in infant-directed speech. *Psychological Science*, 18, 746–751.

Corboz-Warnery, A., Flvaz-Depeursinge, E., Gersch Bettens, C., and Favez, N. (1993). Systemic analysis of father-mother-baby interactions: the Lausanne triadic play. *Infant Mental Health Journal*, 14, 298–316.

Cross, I. (2009). Communicative development: neonate crying reflects patterns of native-language speech. *Current Biology*, 19, R1078–R1079.

Daveson, B., and Kennelly, J. (2000). Music therapy in palliative care for hospitalised children and adolescents. *Journal of Palliative Care.* 16, 35–38.

Dissanayake, E. (2008). If music is the food of love, what about survival and reproductive processes? *Musicae Scientiae*, Special issue, 169–195.

Edwards, J. (1998). Music therapy for children with severe burn injury. *Music Therapy Perspectives*, 16, 20–25.

Edwards, J. (2006). Music therapy in the treatment and management of mental disorders. *Irish Journal of Psychological Medicine*, 23, 33–35.

Edwards, J. (2007). Antecedents of contemporary uses for music in healthcare contexts: the 1890s to the 1940s. In J. Edwards (ed.) *Music: Promoting Health and Creating Community in Healthcare Contexts*, pp. 181–202. (Newcastle upon Tyne: Cambridge Scholars)

Edwards, J. (2011). A music and health perspective on music's perceived 'goodness'. *Nordic Journal of Music Therapy*, 20, 90–101.

Edwards, J., and Kennelly, J. (2011). Music therapy for children in hospital care: a stress and coping framework for practice. In A. Meadows (ed.) *Developments in Music Therapy Practice: Case Perspectives*, pp. 151–165. (Gilsum, NH: Barcelona)

Edwards, J., Scahill, M., and Phelan, H. (2007). Music therapy: promoting healthy mother-infant relations in the vulnerable refugee and asylum seeker community. In J. Edwards (ed.) *Music: Promoting Health and Creating Community*, pp. 154–168. (Newcastle upon Tyne: Cambridge Scholars)

Gerhardt, S. (2004). *Why Love Matters: How Affection Shapes a Baby's Brain.* (London: Routledge)

Gold C., Wigram, T., and Elefant, C. (2006). Music therapy for autistic spectrum disorder (Cochrane Review). *The Cochrane Library*, 2 (Chichester: John Wiley & Sons, Ltd)

Gouk, P. (ed.) (2000). *Musical Healing in Cultural Contexts.* (London: Ashgate)

Ham, J. (2010). *Researching maternal-infant interactions.* Paper presented at the Louis Armstrong Center for Music and Medicine's International Summit (NICU): Rhythm, Breath and Lullaby, Beth Israel Medical Center, New York City, NY.

Ham, J., and Tronick, E. (2009). Relational psychophysiology: lessons from mother-infant physiology esearch on dyadically expanded states of consciousness. *Psychotherapy Research*, 19, 619–632.

Hargreaves, D. (1982). *The Developmental Psychology of Music.* (Cambridge: Cambridge University Press)

Hughes, M. (1995). A comparison of mother-infant interactions and the client-therapist relationship. In A. Wigram, B. Saperston, and R. West (eds) *The Art and Science of Music Therapy: a Handbook*, pp. 296–306. (London: Harwood Academic)

John, D. (1992). Towards music psychotherapy. *British Music Journal of Therapy*, 6, 10–13.

Jonsdottir, V. (2002). Musicking in early intervention. *Voices: a World Forum for Discussion*, 2, np. Available at https://normt.uib.no/index.php/voices/article/viewArticle/86. Accessed December 2010.

Levitin, D., and Rogers. S. (2005). Absolute pitch: perception, coding, and controversies. *Trends in Cognitive Sciences*, 9, 26–33.

Loewy, J.V. (1995). The musical stages of speech: a developmental model of pre-verbal sound making. *Music Therapy*, 13, 47–73.

Mackenzie, J., and Hamlet, K. (2005). The Music Together program: addressing the needs of 'well' families with young children. *Australian Journal of Music Therapy*, 16, 43–56.

MacKinlay, E., and Baker, F. (2005). Nurturing herself, nurturing her baby: creating positive experiences for first-time mothers through lullaby singing. *Women and Music–A Journal of Gender and Culture*, 9, 69–89.

Malloch, S. (1999). Mother and infants and communicative musicality. *Musicae Scientiae*, Special Issue, 13–28.

Malloch, S., and Trevarthen, C. (2008). Musicality: communicating the vitality and interest of life. In S. Malloch, and C. Trevarthen (eds) *Communicative Musicality: Exploring the Basis for Human Companionship*, pp. 1–11. (Oxford: Oxford University Press)

Mampe, B., Friederici, A., Christophe, A., and Wermke, K. (2009). Newborns' cry melody is shaped by their native language. *Current Biology*, 19, 1994–1997.

Maselko, J., Kubzansky, L., Lipsitt, L. and Burka, S. (2010). Mother's affection at 8 months predicts emotional distress in adulthood. *Journal of Epidemiology and Community Health*, np. doi:10.1136/jech.2009.097873.

Miyamoto, K. (2007). Music characteristics of preschool-age students: a review of literature. *UPDATE*, 32, 26–40.

Nakata, T., and Trehub, S. (2004). Infants 'responsiveness to maternal speech and singing. *Infant Behaviour and Development*, 27, 455–464.

Nicholson, J., Berthelsen, D., Abad, V., Williams, K., and Bradley, J. (2008). Impact of music therapy to promote positive parenting and child development. *Journal of Health Psychology*, 13, 226–238.

Noone, J. (2008). Developing a music therapy programme within a person centred planning framework. *Voices: a World Forum for Music Therapy*, 3 np. Available at https://normt.uib.no/index.php/voices/article/view/420. Accessed January 2010.

Oldfield. A. (1995). Music therapy with families. In A. Wigram, B. Saperston, and R. West (eds) *The Art and Science of Music Therapy: a Handbook*, pp. 46–54. (London: Harwood Academic)

Oldfield, A., and Bunce, L. (2001). 'Mummy can play too . . .' - short term music therapy with mothers and young children. *British Journal of Music Therapy*, 15, 27–36.

Oldfield, A., and Flower, C. (2008). *Music Therapy with Children and their Families.* (London: Jessica Kingsley)

O'Neill, C., Trainor, L. J., and Trehub, S. E. (2001). Infants' responsiveness to fathers' singing. *Music Perception*, 18, 409–425.

Oldfield, A., Bunce, L., and Adams, M. (2003). An investigation into short-term music therapy with mothers and young children. *British Journal of Music Therapy*, 17, 26–45.

Papoušek, M. (1996). Intuitive parenting: a hidden source of musical stimulation in infancy. In I. Deliege and J. Sloboda (eds) *Musical Beginnings: Origins and Development of Musical Competence*, pp. 88–112. (Oxford: Oxford University Press)

Pavlicevic, M. (2000). Improvisation in music therapy: human communication in sound. *Journal of Music Therapy*, 37, 269–285.

Plantinga, J., and Trainor, L. (2009). Melody recognition by two month old infants. *Journal of the Acoustical Society of America*, 125, EL58–EEL62.

Raglio, A., Bellelli, G., Traficante, D., Gianotti, M., Ubezio, M., Villani, D., and Trabucchi, M. (2008). Efficacy of music therapy in the treatment of behavioural and psychiatric symptoms of dementia. *Alzheimer's Disease and Associated Disorders*, 22, 158–162.

Robb, L. (1999). Emotional musicality in mothering; vocal affect, and an acoustic study of postnatal depression. *Musicae Scientiae*, Special Issue, 123–154.

Robertson, J. (1953). *A child goes to hospital*. Film. (London: Tavistock Child Development Research Centre)

Schellenberg, G., and Trehub, S. (2003). Good pitch memory is widespread. *Psychological Science*, 14, 262–266.

Schore, A. (2001). The effects of early relational trauma on right brain development, affect attunement, and infant mental health. *Infant Mental Health Journal*, 22, 201–269.

Schore, A. (2009). Relational trauma and the developing right brain: the neurobiology of broken attachment bonds. In T. Baradon (ed.) *Relational Trauma in Infancy*, pp. 19–47. (London: Routledge)

Shoemark, H. (1996). Family-centred early intervention: music therapy in the playgroup program. *Australian Journal of Music Therapy*, 7, 3–15.

Shoemark, H., and Dearn, T. (2008). Keeping the family at the centre of family-centred music therapy with hospitalised infants. *Australian Journal of Music Therapy*, 19, 3–24.

Standley, J., Walworth, D., and Nguyen, J. (2009). Effect of parent/child group music activities on toddler development: a pilot study. *Music Therapy Perspectives*, 27, 11–15.

Stern, D. (1977). *The First Relationship: Infant and Mother*. (Cambridge, MA: Harvard University Press)

Stern, D. (2000). *The Interpersonal World of the Infant: a View from Psychoanalysis and Developmental Psychology*, 2nd Edn. (New York: Karnac Books)

Stewart, K. (2009). Dimensions of the voice: the use of voice and breath with infants and caregivers in the NICU. In R. Azoulay, and J. Loewy (eds) *Music, the Breath, and Health: Advances in Integrative Music Therapy*, pp. 235–250. (New York: Satchnote Press)

Streeter, E. (1999). Finding a balance between psychological thinking and musical awareness in music therapy theory: a psychoanalytic perspective. *British Journal of Music Therapy*, 13, 5–20.

Sullivan J. (2007). Music for the injured soldier: a contribution of American women's military bands during World War II. *Journal of Music Therapy*, 44, 282–305.

Tan, X., Yowler, C., Super, D., and Fratianne, R. (2010). The efficacy of music therapy protocols for decreasing pain, anxiety, and muscle tension levels during burn dressing changes: a prospective randomized crossover trial. *Journal of Burn Care and Research*, 4, 590–597.

Trainor, L. (1996). Infant preferences for infant-directed versus noninfant-directed playsongs and lullalbies. *Infant Behavior and Development*, 19, 83–92.

Trehub, S. (2003). The developmental origins of musicality. *Nature Neuroscience*, 6, 669–673.

Trehub, S., and Trainor, L. (1998). Singing to infants: lullabies and playsongs. *Advances in Infancy Research*, 12, 43–77.

Trehub, S., Trainor, L., and Unyk, A. (1993). Music and speech processing in the first year of life. In H. W. Reese (ed.) *Advances in Child Development and Behaviour*, pp. 1–35. (San Diego, CA: Academic)

Trehub, S., Unyk, A., and Henderson, J. (1994). Children's songs to infant siblings: parallels with speech. *Journal of Child Language*, 21, 735–744.

Trevarthem C. (2001a). Intrinsic motivations for companionship in understanding: their origins, development, and significant for infant mental health. *Infant Mental Health Journal*, 22, 95–131.

Trevarthen, C. (2001b). Infant intersubjectivity: research, theory, and clinical applications. *The Journal of Child Psychology and Psychiatry and Allied Disciplines*, 42, 3–48.

Trolldalen, G. (1997). Music therapy and interplay: a music therapy project with mothers and children elucidated through the concept of 'appreciative recognition'. *Nordic Journal of Music Therapy*, 6, 14–27.

Tsang, C., and Conrad, N, (2010). Does the message matter? The effect of song type on infants' pitch preferences for lullabies and playsongs. *Infant Behavior and Development*, 33, 96–100.

van der Horst, F., and van der Veer, R. (2010). The ontogeny of an idea: John Bowlby and contemporaries on mother-child separation. *History of Psychology*, 13, 25–45.

Volkova, A., Trehub, S.E., and Schellenberg, E.G. (2006). Infants' memory for musical performances. *Developmental Science*, 9, 584–590.

Vosoughi, S., Roy, B., Frank, M., and Roy, D. (2010). Effects of caregiver prosody on child language acquisition. *Speech Prosody*, 100429, 1–4.

Wallin, D. (2007). *Attachment in Psychotherapy*. (London: Guilford Press)

Wermke, K., Mende, W., Manfredi, C., and Bruscaglioni, P. (2002). Developmental aspects of infant's cry melody and formants. *Medical Engineering & Physics*, 24, 501–514.

Winnicott, D.W. (1952). *Through Paediatrics to Psychoanalysis: Collected Papers*. (London: Karnac)

Winnicott, D. (1965). *The Maturational Processes and the Facilitating Environment*. (London: Hogarth Press)

Chapter 2

Becoming in tune: The use of music therapy to assist the developing bond between traumatized children and their new adoptive parents

Tiffany Drake

I was anxious that music therapy would be another place where he could say 'you're not the mother I want'. But over time he . . . allowed me to join in the music. Sometimes he'd say 'stop' and that was OK. I think it taught me to allow him to set the pace with our relationship and not to impose a relationship on him and gradually he trusted me more and more and he began to communicate with me through the music and not just in his own little world so I think some of the walls between us came down.

A mother's reflection on participating in music therapy with her adopted son.

Finding the pulse
Chaos . . . Noise . . . Disorder . . .

This is often my first impression of the music of adopted and traumatized children beginning music therapy. In these early sessions, as I briefly meet the child and explore the quality of their developing relationship with their adoptive parent, their behaviour can appear unregulated and erratic and they may present with heightened anxiety. This may be evident through avoidant, controlling or withdrawn behaviours. Achieving a musical connection can feel like a daunting task. This struggle can provide me with a flavour of the experience of the parents trying to get to know their adopted child, who might frequently resist their attempts at contact, avoiding communication. A child might explore the music therapy room with great energy, for example, but with fleeting strikes of various instruments as they dash from one thing to another, making it impossible to 'capture' any of their music, or to hold them within even the shortest of musical exchanges. The experience reminds me that the adoptive parents have not had the chance to hold, cradle and nurture this child as a babe-in-arms and how the child has learnt, possibly through being neglected or experiencing negative physical contact, to avoid such holding and to survive alone without it. This pervasive loss is frequently evident from my first contact with these fragile and fragmented children and their often struggling, but determined and committed new parents.

In such a chaotic introduction there is little room for words. Words may have been experienced as threatening, abusive and even dangerous by some of these adopted children. While words give the adult some degree of control, engaging verbally is sometimes too risky for children who may have previously experienced interactions with adults as abusive or neglectful. Verbal children might try to avoid forming a musical connection with me by talking constantly as they play the instruments. Non-verbal children may vocalize loud utterances that punctuate their chaotic playing. Highly anxious children may ask many questions such as 'who do the instruments belong to?' and 'what do the instruments do?' but they seldom wait for answers, instead filling any potential space with more questions or sounds.

This chaotic behaviour is the child's means of controlling an uncertain and unknown environment. It enables them to repeatedly avoid or break any potential contact. Their experience of forming relationships has often been characterized by inconsistency, disruption, negativity and abuse. Chaos and destruction therefore become their way of surviving, controlling, or avoiding new relationships. Repeated negative experience builds fear and mistrust, even of positive interactions, and teaches the child that it is safer to disrupt a potential relationship than to engage in it, only to risk being hurt or disappointed again. Music therapy can provide an environment for these children to explore positive and creative connections with others, gradually mitigating their disrupted patterns of emotions and responses.

From chaos to order

I am presented with many challenges each time I meet a new family referred for music therapy by Coram's Adoption and Permanent Families Service. Coram offers a range of services to families, including hosting the third largest

independent adoption agency in the UK. The children placed for adoption by
the service have all experienced traumatic starts in life. They are likely to have
experienced abuse or neglect, disrupted early relationships and multiple foster
placements. Many were born to drug or alcohol addicted mothers or to women
with mental health difficulties.

Music therapy is the beginning of a journey by which it is hoped that the
chaos may transform into attunement (Stern 1985), and the disorder become
harmony between parent and child. This journey is made possible through co-
improvised music which 'can be a productive, safe way of expressing, organising
and containing the dynamic ebb and flow of moment-by-moment shifts in
feeling and experience' (Stewart 1996 p. 21). It is anticipated that the therapy
will help the child to begin to trust the parent to respond to them with love and
offer them security. Finding the rhythm to which child and parent can move
together requires that I relinquish my musical expectations and find the basic
pulse to which their relationship can become attuned. These initial moments
of connection may be almost imperceptible at first but enable both child and
adoptive parent a moment of shared creativity which may begin to change the
former's damaged attachment pattern (Robarts 2009).

Almost 50% of children placed by Coram are adopted before 3 years of age.
The children may have developmental and/or learning difficulties. The impact
of traumatic experience results in hyperarousal or dissociated behaviours
(Perry et al. 1995). Early trauma can impact right-hemisphere brain development (Schore 2001), the sphere responsible for socio-emotional information
and empathy (Schore 2001; Gerhardt 2004; Panksepp and Trevarthen 2009) as
well as for musical appreciation and expression (Panksepp and Trevarthen
2009). A traumatic early start has already had a damaging effect on the child's
attachment relationships and emotional well-being and will have compromised their ability to develop resilience, self-esteem, concentration, regulation
and sense of identity. There is increasing evidence of the long-term impact of
abusive, neglectful or disrupted early relationships and the need to intervene as
early as possible to ensure that any disturbance is mitigated before becoming
set (Baradon et al. 2005).

Many of the children Coram supports display affection indiscriminately as
the lack of a consistent attachment figure precludes the development of
stranger wariness. They may also be impulsive in their behaviour or show
intense emotional responses through lack of self-regulation. They are likely to
have what are described as 'disorganised attachments' (Gerhardt 2004; Prior
and Glaser 2006). These are typified by a lack of coherent behaviours in
responding to separation from the attachment figure evident in contradictory
behavioural patterns, for example, strong attachment behaviour then sudden

avoidance, mistimed movements and expressions, disorientation or rapid changes in affect (Prior and Glaser 2006) and fear of the attachment figure leading to confusion of fear and love (Gerhardt 2004). With this confused background, the love of a nurturing adoptive family alone may not be enough to give the adopted child a better outlook for the future and many of these children will need additional support such as some form of therapy (Lush et al. 1998).

In addition to the needs of the child, the therapist must be aware that adoptive parents may have their own experiences of grief and loss such as living with infertility, having prior experience of miscarriage(s), bereavement, or stillborn babies before proceeding with the psychologically and emotionally demanding process of adopting. The adoptive parent or couple's responses to their own experiences of loss therefore forms part of the milieu in which the therapy for such families takes place.

Where a child's background is particularly complex or traumatic, music therapy may be offered within weeks of a child's placement to a family to assist them in bonding together. Sometimes the challenges become apparent some months into placement and music therapy may be offered at this later stage. There can also be key times when emotional or behavioural difficulties arise, such as around transitions to nursery or school, a family bereavement, or the arrival of a newly adopted sibling in the home. At these times a music therapy referral may be warranted. A shared, creative experience in music therapy can allow parent(s) and the child a space to engage in positive play giving them the chance to explore and build a new relationship or to express a range of emotions, fears or anxieties that they cannot put into words.

The parents and child may need support in 'claiming' one another in these fragile early stages of getting to know one another and developing a relationship of trust. Music therapy may provide a safe environment to facilitate this process, not least because of its reliance on musical rather than verbal communication. Within this environment they can learn about one another and develop responsive intimacy, such as takes place within healthily developing relationships (H. Papoušek 1996).

The phenomenon of infant-directed speech or 'motherese', where the mother adapts her speech, pitch, timing and prosody to connect with and respond to her pre-verbal infant, is intrinsic to relating in the early years (M. Papoušek 1996; Mazokopaki and Kugiumutzakis 2009). This responsive musical communication may not have been experienced by neglected infants who have not had a consistent attachment figure. The role of motherese in being sensitive to, and helping to regulate, emotional states (Marwick and Murray 2009) is indicative of its importance in the child's developing capacity for emotional regulation, stability and resilience. Given that adopted children are likely to have experienced trauma and disruption in their lives at a pre-verbal age, they would not have had the developmental competence to put words to their experiences, therefore further compounding the 'non-linguistic' nature of the manifestation of trauma (De Zulueta 1993).

The role of music therapy in supporting parent–child bonding

Early parent–infant communication is intrinsically musical (Malloch 1999; Trevarthen 1999; Trevarthen and Malloch 2002) and this musical relating develops the bonds of relationship (H. Papoušek 1996; M. Papoušek 1996; Pavlicevic 1997; Drake 2008). Music can therefore be used effectively to allow a parent and child, who have not shared this early developmental relating, the chance to experience shared connectedness through musical play.

Lack of sensitive timing in the early musical duet between baby and mother, such as delayed, aggressive, avoidant or intrusive responses, can result in distress, tension and anxiety on the part of the baby even at 2 months of age (Trevarthen 1979; Murray and Andrews 2005). This is indicative of the strong link between interpersonal communication and subjective emotional states (Trevarthen 1979). Children placed for adoption may never have experienced well-attuned, containing mother–infant interaction, a vital pre-cursor to speech, emotional expression and regulation (Fahlberg 1994). Deprivation of such engagement can result in communication, attachment, cognitive and/or emotional difficulties in the child (Murray 1992; Murray et al. 1996; Trevarthen 1999; Drake 2008). Longitudinal studies have shown that hostile interactions by depressed mothers towards their infants in the first few months of life predicts dysregulated behaviour, conduct disorder and hyperactivity at 1, 5, and 8 years of age (Murray et al. 2001; Morrell and Murray 2003; Marwick and Murray 2009).

The absence of an attachment figure, with whom the infant can experience playful, attuned and responsive social communication in the first year of life, may result in delayed development of early communication and relationship behaviours by the infant (Falhberg 1994). When the child's intuitive initiation of communication goes unnoticed, through lack of mirroring and imitation, their desire to connect with another is not fulfilled as they fail to find a partner in their dance.

Music therapy can facilitate this attuned exchange, even at later stages of development, for both parties in the dance. Music may 'permit regression to early, infantile modes of feeling, thinking and meaning' (Stewart 1996 p. 22) and may 'reach into the realm of the pre-verbal self, where it can work on creating deeply rooted creative-constructive change in impaired attachment patterns' (Robarts 2009: p. 383). Where adoptive parents have had a positive model of attachment themselves the phenomenon of musical mother–infant communication may come naturally to them. However, there may be some inhibition in responding in this animated way to a child who is no longer a baby, whereas a baby is born with an innate motivation to invite such interaction. The child may have to 'relearn' how to engage in social exchanges in a playful, communicative and well-attuned way, first by developing a basic trust that the adult will respond to them in these positive ways. This may take many months of consistent nurturing attention to enable the child to eventually rework internal models of attachment.

The music therapist may take on the role of supporting the parent in mirroring their child's communication and expression. This can be done through modelling (Drake 2008; Salkeld 2008; Wigram and Elefant 2009) rather than giving verbal direction, which might feel persecutory to the 'new' parent. I have found that attempting to understand the child's experiences of relationships, particularly their internal model of attachment, is necessary to best support them in therapy. Where their prior experiences have been traumatic these may need to be re-enacted in some form in the therapy process and may need to be contained and re-worked to enable healthy processing and to facilitate new models of attachment being developed.

Survival and control

Often adopted children have had to learn to survive alone very early in life. Their experiences have taught them that adults cannot be relied upon to meet even their most basic needs. Children who have younger siblings have often become carers to them, even when they are still in infancy themselves, immediately propelling them into adult roles and denying them their own childhood. The child's basic survival instinct, the factor underpinning attachment, is heightened and trust in adults is lost, resulting in a position of total independence in the child (Falhberg 1994). This can be evident in avoidant and defensive behaviours, even in the young infant who turns his head to avoid the gaze of a potentially threatening parent.

A newly adopted child attending music therapy may present with adult concerns. For example, they might ask where I sleep, assuming that I live in the music therapy room but noting that there is no bed present. Frequently they need to be in control as feeling out of control has been experienced as dangerous, threatening or overwhelming. They may present as over-competent with self-parenting behaviours and resist any 'parenting' care or attention offered by the adults in the room, be it from the music therapist or their adoptive parent.

These responses have been learnt as survival mechanisms and the shift in being able to trust others needs to happen at a pace that the child can manage, and often, that they perceive to be in control of themselves. Premature adoption of adult roles can be evident in children who have experienced some kind of trauma and make it difficult for the child to assume age-appropriate behaviours again (Yule et al. 1999).

Children with disorganized attachments in infancy are likely to display controlling behaviour in later childhood (Prior and Glaser 2006). Studies have also found that:

> ...children disorganised in infancy draw a picture of later childhood as being characterised by controlling, angry, hostile and oppositional behaviours. Alongside this external expression of difficulty, however, the studies also indicate that the children are low in self-confidence and social competence, struggling in their academic performance and, in assessments of internal representations, depict the self and caregivers as both frightening and unpredictable or frightened and helpless. (Prior and Glaser 2006 p. 176)

Most of the children referred to me for music therapy are under 5 years of age and frequently this pattern of behaviour and presentation is already beginning to emerge. It is intended that by addressing these issues as early as possible it will ensure a more hopeful prognosis for their future.

These issues of control can make responses to any boundaries set by adults extremely difficult for the child to manage. In music therapy, even the 'Hello' and 'Goodbye' songs, which I use to mark the opening and conclusion of each session, become a threat to be avoided. The response to the first hearing of a greeting song with a newly referred child often gives me insight into their emotional state and their ability to manage adult-imposed structure and boundaries. The child might rush into the room and begin playing and talking to avoid my setting of the beginning of the session. This can result in the greeting song not being possible. If we do manage to sing the song the child often becomes very withdrawn during this positive attention as though the experience is overwhelming. They may become angry towards me or their parent, or, conversely, cling to their parent avoiding eye contact as they hide their head in the parent's chest or clothing. While this may sound indicative of a close relationship where the child is appropriately seeking protection or safety with the parent it can also show the child's fragility and vulnerability and their confusion at the opportunity for intimacy. Some children's response to changes in attachment figures is to become overly clingy and dependent (Falhberg 1994) as in Sam's story below.

The challenge of separation: Sam and May

Sam appeared to have bonded well with his adoptive parents, May and Richard, when placed with them at 2 years of age. However, after living with them for

6 months, he had become very clingy with May. He was incredibly anxious when visitors came to the house and would not let go of May. This also made leaving the house very difficult as Sam was inseparable from her. His parents became particularly concerned when Sam also stopped crying at these times of apparent fear and distress as though too consumed by his anxiety to do so. Often families are referred by Coram's Adoption Service for music therapy to assist with the formation of an affectionate and secure bond. In this instance Sam needed to develop his security and self-confidence to enable him to survive separation from May in a healthy, resilient way.

In his first music therapy session Sam remained physically attached to May and barely uttered a sound. May and Richard, along with their social worker, had described to me that Sam's language development was delayed and that, although he was now 2½ years old, he showed no signs of beginning to speak. He eyed me cautiously from his mother's lap and only tapped at the drum tentatively after a great deal of encouragement from her. As Sam became more familiar with me and the music therapy room, over subsequent weeks, he began to explore some of the instruments which were placed a little distance from May's lap.

Sam was fascinated by the large, low, floor drum. His first significant separation from May was to clamber up onto it and, barely before he was stood up on it, to jump off into May's lap. This tentative exploration of separation indicated a distorted sense of time that is common in adopted and fostered children (Jackson 2004). The use of a steady rhythm might help to develop this 'game' which, at this stage, lacked any element of playfulness, into a useful way to increase Sam's ability to separate from May. Over the following weeks Sam continued to explore being apart from May through jumping off the drum into her lap. His urgency to be reunited with her meant that, initially, he struggled to engage with the anticipation of a 'ready, steady, . . . [go]' type cue. Sam repeated the game over and over again as though testing his own capacity to engage in it. Little by little he was able to wait longer before jumping, surviving a tiny bit more time in separation from her.

During this phase games of peekaboo also began to emerge in Sam's play. This game is more normally associated with infants from around 6 months of age and plays a role in supporting their developing social awareness as well as facilitating social and emotional co-regulation through balanced repetition and variation (Gratier and Apter-Danon 2009). Timing and anticipation are crucial to the game with mid-range predictability providing the greatest enjoyment to the infant (Fernald and O'Neil 1993; Gratier and Apter-Danon 2009). For Sam it appeared to be part of his developmental process of surviving separation from May and trusting that she would still be there after a brief absence.

A lack of anticipation and expectation was also evident in this play but gradually Sam could tolerate the waiting a little more before his mother reappeared. This was assisted by a musical framework to help reduce any anxiety during the period of absence as the music indicated that something still 'existed' rather than Sam being left with the void created by silence, even despite the implication of anticipation that the game itself creates. Sam's emotional response to these games was serious and earnest rather than playful. My musical accompaniment to them and May's lively and animated engagement reassured Sam of the playful element, however, and gradually there were flickers of a smile or a glint in his eye as his mother announced her reappearance from behind a lollipop drum. There was a gradual shift from the purposeful to the playful. Through consistent repetition Sam grew to trust that May would always be there again for him and allowed himself to experience the playful elements in the game.

From Session 7, as he appeared to be more settled in the setting, we began to introduce Sam to the idea of May being absent from the music therapy room. She explained to Sam that she needed to go to the toilet and would be back very soon. He was involved in playing with a basket of mixed small percussion with me and continued to engage in this, exploring the different instruments, until May returned a few minutes later. He looked at her and smiled. At the end of this session he hid in the instrument cupboard, as though recalling the separation. May and I sang to him during this hiding game to reassure Sam that we had him in mind until he was ready to be found by May again after a few moments. His little smile on being 'found' began to reassure May that he trusted her to be there for him again after a brief period of separation.

Over the remaining 12 weeks of therapy May left the room for gradually increasing periods. Sam was able to survive these and found appropriate strategies to reassure himself that she would return, such as choosing three matching instruments for us to play, one symbolizing May in her absence. Once he stood on the floor drum again and said 'Mama', wanting to jump into the safety of her lap. I explained that she was coming back soon and that he could jump to me. He paused. With building anticipation I sang 'ready, steady, . . .' and off he jumped into my lap, giggling with delight and surprise at the risk he had taken. Sam was becoming more confident in himself. This was evident as his music became more sustained and he was able to take his own role in little duets and trios that we could play together. His sense of shared timing was clearly developing as he could engage with a steady rhythmic pulse. Having his musical contributions reflected and mirrored helped to assure Sam of the value of his independent role in our mutual creativity. His speech also developed, particularly in the home environment where his parents reported him using three- and four-word sentences. He was sometimes even brave enough to use words to make choices in the therapy room.

By the end of his music therapy Sam was able to stay in the room for whole sessions without May present, much to her and Richard's amazement. May always joined us for the 'Goodbye' song as a safe way for them to be reunited before the journey home and so that Sam could share with her things that he had been doing in the session. By this stage May described Sam as 'chatty' and this was becoming true in my presence too as he talked excitedly about the instruments and what we would play together.

Music therapy sessions allowed Sam and May to engage in games more readily associated with younger infants as part of an attachment relationship, despite the fact that they had not been part of the same family at that time. The games served a developmental purpose for Sam in his attachment process as they would for a younger child in the birth family. This 'revisiting' of play and behaviours from a younger chronological age can be given an age-appropriate context when supported by music and is a frequent occurrence in my experience of working with adoptive families.

Repeatedly exploring separation through symbolic play and actions assisted Sam in trusting May to provide a 'secure base' from which he could explore (Bowlby 1988) rather than needing to constantly cling to her for fear of losing her otherwise. The musical underpinning, often only the 'secure base' of a steady pulse, enabled Sam to develop a more coherent sense of internal timing through which this exploration could take place. It also provided a sense of consistency and reassurance enabling Sam to take risks within the musical context rather than stepping out into a silent void. The musical accompaniment assured him that he was still held in mind and not abandoned to explore alone.

The challenge of rejection: Charlie and Ruth

Unlike Sam, 4-year-old Charlie did not develop a clinging bond to his adoptive mother Ruth. Conversely, she described struggling to bond with Charlie while he appeared to bond with his adoptive father, Peter. Ruth here describes her journey with Charlie and the role of music therapy in nurturing their relationship.[1]

After a few months of having Charlie live with us we were really struggling – in a sense we were on our knees emotionally. Charlie was showing us lots of anxiety and pushing boundaries and

---

[1] The text that appears in italics here is taken from an interview with Ruth conducted for the making of a short film *When Words Are Not Enough* about Coram's Music Therapy Service in 2007 by D. Francis (filmmaker, editor and producer).

seemed unhappy which was devastating for him and for us. The hard days were more common than the good days. We were dealing with a child who was grieving for his foster family. Charlie bonded with my husband and not with me. I think the level of anxiety in me about 'am I ever going to bond with this child' was in some way communicated to Charlie.

Ruth described Charlie as being very afraid of noise, saying he would freeze or panic at loud noises and once pleaded with her to stop dancing and singing along to the radio. She also described how he needed to be in control and appeared afraid if he felt out of control. This made the situation at home very challenging. Ruth goes on to explain how they came to music therapy.

Our social worker thought that music therapy for me and Charlie together might be a way to explore how to be a mother and son. Music therapy was amazing. It was helpful for me and my husband to meet the music therapist first and talk with her on our own to learn a bit about music therapy and let her hear why we were in the crisis we were in.

Our experience of the sessions was extraordinary. It immediately felt safe – for Charlie there was a welcome and sense it was about him. At first I wondered if he was going to make use of them because he just seemed to make a lot of noise and be quite uncommunicative. He was needing to be in control of things and say 'is this place safe for me' but the therapist was so affirming that he was able to express some of his anxieties and lay them down, sometimes quite literally.

In one session Charlie built an enormous tower-like structure out of all the instruments. Ruth and I wondered what he was going to do with this structure when suddenly he began to destroy it *'letting the mess cascade around us'*. Ruth described this point in the therapy as:

. . . a watershed time where he let me into the mess – it felt like a huge step of trust for him to say 'I know you're going to be there for me, I know it's OK to show you when I'm sad or angry or just don't understand and that I need you' and there is something in us as parents that we need to know that. He showed us the distress and confusion inside himself and found a language to let it out. He learnt that he doesn't have to cope with things on his own.

I was anxious that music therapy would be another place where he could say 'you're not the mother I want'. But over time he gradually allowed me to join in the music. Sometimes he'd say 'stop' and that was OK. I think it taught me to allow him to set the pace with our relationship and not to impose a relationship on him and gradually he trusted me more and more and he began to communicate with me through the music and not just in his own little world so I think some of the walls between us came down.

As a prospective adoptive mother, as I was then, there was a huge relief that 'I'm able to communicate with this child and he's able to communicate with me and he wants to'. For me, some of those fears whether Charlie would allow me to be his mum went through music therapy in ways that I couldn't have anticipated.

I think that [music therapy] has made a huge difference to Charlie. He's much happier. He found a way to let all that was bubbling away inside out and sometimes that was very frightening for him – watching his level of anger. [But] he's learned an emotional language that he simply didn't have before and I think learning it without words was very helpful for him.

We just love him, but we certainly needed help to learn to love him in a way he could receive and I think that's what music therapy has done for us. He's just such a happy little boy. He's much more our child now rather than 'daddy's' child and the bond between him and me is very close – I think because we had that experience of doing music therapy together – just the two of us. Music therapy [gave us] a wonderful journey of hope.

Within the safety of the therapeutic space Charlie was able to share his grief, distress and anxiety and to allow Ruth to witness it. This process of 'showing' something of the internal world to the attachment figure is an important step in the developing bond of trust. Doing this within the safety of a therapeutic space allowed Charlie to test Ruth's capacity to survive what felt so threatening to him, with me as a third party witness and support for each of them. This, in turn, gave Ruth the 'permission' to help him manage his internal 'mess' as he let her in to his sense of grief and chaos. The chaos and destruction could begin to be replaced by the possibility of engaging in a positive experience of mutual creativity through making music together. The impact of this was evident in Charlie's increasingly coherent music and shared duets as the chaos became manageable with the support and containment of his mother.

For some children these steps have to be taken in a more tentative manner to ensure the child feels safe in sharing their vulnerability. Where human relationships are still perceived as potentially threatening or untrustworthy a child may feel safer exploring responses through explorative play or by removing feelings and experiences to a safe distance as though to test them out before committing themselves to the risk of direct human contact.

Displacement: Matthew

Matthew, aged 3, had experienced many separations due to several foster placements and periods with his birth parents before being placed with his adoptive family. This pattern of loss meant that goodbyes and endings filled him with anxiety and distress. In music therapy Matthew did all he could to prolong the session to avoid the ending. Whenever I mentioned that we had to prepare to say goodbye he would become very withdrawn and distressed. He was a child with language delay but his vocal expression would regress even further at the idea of the ending as he would whimper and moan as though fearful of the separation. At these times Matthew found direct personal contact very challenging. His distress could be gently alleviated by feeling it was shared and acknowledged. My attempts to do this directly were too overwhelming for him, however, reminding me that he may not have experienced contingent or containing emotional responses in his early life.

Matthew was fond of the teddy bear which lived on the windowsill in the music therapy room. During one difficult transition to the 'Goodbye' song I picked up the bear and said that I thought he didn't like goodbyes either and found it really hard to say goodbye. From the corner of the room, where Matthew sat slumped with his head in his arms, I heard a little voice say 'yeah'. He lifted his head and looked at the bear. I focused on the bear and said 'you don't like goodbyes either do you Bear, but we do need to sing goodbye to each other until we do music again next week'. Matthew jumped up and rushed towards me, bear and the piano and said 'OK, c'mon bear' and sat down on the stool next to me. He held the bear's paw and with his other hand tapped along at the piano as we sang the song.

Removing the directness of the goodbye from me to the safety of the toy bear enabled Matthew to know that his feelings were shared in a non-threatening way. The bear had identified with him, enabling him to take the responsibility of identifying with the bear. This method of displacement can assist children in finding creative ways through challenging moments and overwhelming feelings as it enables them to be managed but at a safe distance (Rustin 1999). This approach is also evident for children who use storytelling as part of their therapeutic process to convey feelings or experiences as the world of fantasy and reality can be merged.

Storytelling as a music therapy technique

In music therapy sessions stories may be elaborated and given additional dramatic effect to convey the emotions children are exploring by using instruments to create the 'sound world' of the story. For adopted children, creating stories in the third person enables them to share aspects about their experiences consciously or unconsciously in a safer way than directly referring to people or experiences in their past (Salkeld 2008). The story stem technique has been used as a model of evaluating adoptive children's internal working models of attachment and how these evolve through their placement (Hodges et al. 2003). This technique uses displacement to allow children to represent their experiences in a safely removed way.

The story stem starts with a set-up using dolls or toys that are not representative of the child's family such as the tale of a piglet who has wandered away from his pig sty past the other animals and gets lost. The researcher asks the child to show and tell her what happens next in the story. Typically, by way of example, securely attached children might say that the mummy pig realizes the piglet is missing and goes to look for him and finds him to bring him safely home. An insecurely attached child, however, may complete the story with a disastrous scenario in which the pig is attacked by other animals or lost forever in the woods and no one comes to look for him and his mummy, if he has one, does not even notice he is lost.

Musical stories: Sara and John

Sara was 3 years old when she began music therapy. She had been in her adoptive placement for about 2 months. As a child who had cared for younger siblings in her birth home she displayed adult concerns and frequently took on adult responsibilities as though not trusting adults to assume these roles. She was verbally eloquent and bright for her age. In many ways this presented her with some challenges as she sought to make intellectual sense of the changes that had occurred in her life. Her adoptive parents were struggling to manage her extreme changes in mood and emotional outbursts. She was very rejecting towards her main carer, her adoptive father, John, and it was decided that music therapy might assist them in bonding.

From her second session Sara began telling the story of a cow. This story then lasted several months until she found some resolution which reflected her changing sense of security and developing attachment with her new parents.

Sara would prompt me to sing by telling me phrases from the story as I reflected the feelings in my piano accompaniment. John usually played various percussion instruments to accompany the story, sometimes with non-verbal indications from Sara controlling his playing and when he should stop. Sara played a duck whistle which she used to emulate the cow's mooing in a very expressive manner. She played this sitting huddled over a small table with her back to John. Sara seemed to offer small elements of the developing story as though to test our capacity to cope with its themes of sadness, loss and abandonment. This showed her adult concern of assessing whether we could manage the challenges of the story in our role as witnesses to her traumatic experiences rather than becoming overwhelmed by it ourselves.

Initially the cow was alone in the field with no one to hear him mooing. Sara said he felt sad and was all alone; no one would come to help him. He then wanted milk but there was no one to bring it to him. Then he stopped mooing because he was too sad to moo any more. Eventually, in an act of determination and resilience, he tries again and again and again to moo but still nobody comes. The sense of loneliness and desolation in the story was almost overwhelming as Sara wanted me and John to witness and share in her own feelings of isolation and neglect.

Over the weeks the story would take strange turns. Once the farmer heard the cow and was going to bring some milk but then seemed to disappear.

Random characters would appear and take the cow to other places suddenly. The cow then appeared to settle more in one place. He could moo again and then, finally, the farmer heard him. Soon the farmer not only brought him milk when he was thirsty but also began to play and dance and sing with the cow. The sparse, melancholic music transformed into playful dancing melodies accompanied by lively rhythms from John on percussion and light joyful mooing from Sara as she jigged about the room.

The reflection of the baby wanting milk and not having her cries responded to in Sara's story may have been true of her own experience as a neglected infant. The 'stopping mooing' reminded me of neglected babies that cease to cry after some time of learning that crying does not illicit a response, such as in poor institutionalized care (Drake 2008). The different characters seemed to reflect social workers and the myriad foster placements Sara had experienced. Then finally the cow's needs were met, as Sara's had been in her adoptive placement. Better still, the relationship had become one of playfulness and spontaneity as well as security as she began to allow herself to both imagine and desire playfulness first through the displacement of the story and then in reality by giving John consent to engage with her playfully in their music making.

As the story began to find some resolution so John and Sara's relationship began to shift. She trusted him to play along with the story in his own way and became less directive of his playing. They became more mutual partners in the development of the music supporting the story. Soon after it was given a satisfactory ending and no longer needed to be told repeatedly as she explored her situation and her past. New music could now emerge in our sessions to reaffirm this evolving positive relationship and without Sara always needing to be in control of the themes of our improvisations.

Separation and loss: hide and seek

Such themes of separation, loss and loneliness enacted in Sara's story are common in adopted children's music therapy and may be played out in a variety of ways. One common means of exploring separation and loss in therapy is through behavioural and symbolic representation of these experiences in games of hide-and-seek, as mentioned in the case of Sam above. This play fulfils the role of testing and proving that the adult(s) can hold the child in mind when they are 'absent'. It provides exploration of the developing relationship of trust, and enables developmental games of peekaboo, which the pair may not have experienced together at the appropriate age when such games would have traditionally been played between a caregiver and baby.

Jackson (2004) described the role of hide-and-seek play in psychotherapy with a multiply traumatized adopted little girl. In one instance she made him hide but then got on with another activity herself, failing to find him as though to give him 'a taste of what it might be like to feel abandoned, rejected and tantalized' (Jackson 2004 p. 63). Winnicott (1990) also described how a child might establish 'a private self that is not communicating, and at the same time wanting to communicate and to be found. It is a sophisticated game of hide-and-seek in which *it is a joy to be hidden but disaster not to be found.*' (Winnicott 1990 p. 186).

Being found: Ella and Carrie

A child who suddenly feels out of control in the therapy space may take control again by announcing 'let's play hide-and-seek'. This was the case with 4-year-old Ella, who frequently did this several weeks into her music therapy, once she felt safe enough to take the risk of hiding. She could repeat the game many times within one session and week after week. Primarily she hid and told me and her adoptive mother, Carrie, to look for her. She did not allow us to find her, how-ever, rather wanting to take this responsibility herself, appearing suddenly from her hiding place. She often hid inside the large instrument cupboard and if we knocked on the door or opened it she would cry 'I'm not here, you can't find me' and pull the door shut on herself again. This left Carrie and me to experience the anxiety of when Ella would appear again and our own sense of being abandoned as our looking was rendered useless.

I was aware of my role in Ella's game but also in being with Carrie through the enforced feelings of abandonment. I would sing simple 'looking' songs both to reassure Carrie we would continue being there for Ella until such point where she could accept this, and to give Ella musical cues as to when she might reappear. In the early weeks she seemed either oblivious to the musical phrases which invited her to be found again, instead appearing at times which dis-rupted the song such as mid-phrase. As she became more able to tolerate shared control she would push open the door to be found, grinning, at an appropriate point of anticipation in the song. This demonstrated her ability to allow me and Carrie to become more empathic and involved in Ella's play and that the music could offer her the safety of a clear framework to begin doing this.

Ella could not take the risk of not being found by the mother she was still learning to trust. Instead she maintained control of the 'game' and of her pri-vate, coping self by instructing us not to find her so that she could appear at the moment of her choosing, thereby taking the role of both adult and child in the game. The game lacked the normal intuitive timing of a well-attuned game of peekaboo between mother and infant.

Ella's game developed and evolved as she was able to explore 'being found' by her new mother in ways which symbolized her adoption more graphically.

She instructed her mother that she was being a stone or a statue and that Carrie had to bring her to life. This could be done by gentle stroking or by playful tickling. In other games she would take on the role of being a baby that Carrie had to mother, nurture, feed, play with and, significantly, find and name as the baby was lost and nameless. The play seemed to let Carrie know how much Ella needed to be claimed by this new mother. Through the play Ella could become a spontaneous, feeling and communicating individual within their developing relationship.

This searching for affirmation of identity is a common process in therapy whereby child and parent explore how to be together simultaneously. My role in this process, as the journey unfolds, shifts from one of facilitation through to support and finally one of observation.

Conclusion

Over the weeks or months of music therapy with these dyads I become the observer to their developing harmony as the chaos and noise gradually and subtly merges into a tuneful, ordered and fluid musical connection. Once a strong and stable connection is established between child and parent they no longer need my role as enabler or holder and I become redundant in the room. The experience of becoming surplus to requirements is an exciting one as the journey in the therapy room comes to an end. The journey then continues outside for this new family without the necessity of my support once they have found and claimed one another.

Intervention in the case of attachment difficulties and disorders often focuses on addressing the capacity for sensitivity and responsiveness in the caregiver (Prior and Glaser 2006). The children I have described above are all fortunate to have been placed within families of wonderfully supportive and giving parents whose sole desire is to create a safe, loving and nurturing home for these vulnerable and grieving children. Sometimes additional support is needed for these children to develop a secure base from which they can trust their new parents, and to establish the sense of security that enables them to know that they will be safely protected and loved unconditionally in this 'forever family'.

Music therapy can offer a safe and consistent space in which to explore and develop the capacity for relationship for damaged and fragile children. The therapeutic relationship creates a triangle of support within which the parent–child relationship can be tested with less risk of betrayal, disruption, or aban-donment. The music can provide a stable base which can affirm the presence of consistent support and additionally assist in developing the capacity for playfulness, spontaneity, and creativity both in the child and between parent and child. This allows them to find a shared rhythm and means of creative expression and communication without the need for words, and for those aspects of relating that words are unable to express.

Allowing an adoptive child a safe place for exploration and sharing of their fears, grief, anxieties, and traumas without the threat or demands that words might evoke can give them the resilience to risk placing trust in others. Going back to the beginnings of a nurturing relationship through shared pre-verbal social communication, typified by exchanges in rhythm, pitch, and timing, enables the pair to find a shared music and the security of a steady pulse on which the stable foundation of their communication and relationship might develop and ultimately rest. For the vast majority of infants growing up in the context of their birth family this is the most natural unconscious process between baby and mother. For those whose early relationships have been disrupted, finding a shared musical language may take a more elaborated, patient, and professional process of help.

References

Baradon, T., Broughton, C., Gibbs, I., James, J., Joyce, A., and Woodhead, J. (2005). *The Practice of Psychoanalytic Parent-Infant Psychotherapy*. (London: Routledge)

Bowlby, J. (1988). *A Secure Base: Clinical Applications of Attachment Theory*. (London: Routledge)

De Zulueta, F. (1993). *From Pain to Violence*. (London: Whurr)

Drake, T. (2008). Back to basics: community-based music therapy for vulnerable young children and their parents. In A. Oldfield, and C. Flower (eds) *Music Therapy with Children and their Families*, pp. 37–52. (London: Jessica Kingsley)

Fahlberg. V. (1994). *A Child's Journey through Placement*. (London: British Association for Adoption and Fostering)

Fernald, A., and O'Neil, D. (1993). Peekaboo across cultures: how mothers and infants play with voices, faces and expectations. In K. MacDonald, and A.D. Pellegrini (eds) *Parent-Child Play: Descriptions and Implications*, pp. 259–286. (Albany, NY: SUNY)

Gerhardt, S. (2004). *Why Love Matters*. (East Sussex: Routledge)

Gratier, M., and Apter-Danon, G. (2009). The improvised musicality of belonging: repetition and variation in mother-infant vocal interaction. In S. Malloch, and C. Trevarthen (eds) *Communicative Musicality*, pp. 301–330. (Oxford: OUP)

Hodges J., Steele, M., Hillman, S., Henderson, K., and Kanuik, J. (2003). Changes in attachment representations over the first year of adoptive placement: narratives of maltreated children. *Clinical Child Psychology and Psychiatry*, 8, 347–363.

Jackson, E. (2004). Trauma revisited: a 5-year-old's journey from experiences, to thoughts, to words, towards hope. *Journal of Child Psychology*, 30, 53–70.

Lush, D., Boston, M., Morgan, J., and Kolvin, I. (1998). Psychoanalytic psychotherapy with disturbed adopted and foster children: a single case follow-up study. *Clinical Child Psychology and Psychiatry*, 3, 51–69.

Malloch, S. (1999). Mother and infants and communicative musicality. *Musicae Scientiae*, Special Issue, 29–57.

Marwick, H., and Murray, L. (2009). The effects of maternal depression on the 'musicality' of infant-directed speech and conversational engagement. In S. Malloch, and C. Trevarthen (eds) *Communicative Musicality*, pp. 281–300. (Oxford: OUP)

Mazokopaki, K., and Kugiumutzakis, G. (2009). Infant rhythms: expressions of musical companionship. In S. Malloch, and C. Trevarthen (eds) *Communicative Musicality*, pp.185–208. (Oxford: OUP)

Morrell, J., and Murray, L. (2003). Postnatal depression and the development of conduct disorder and hyperactive symptoms in childhood: a prospective longitudinal study from 2 months to 8 years. *Journal of Child Psychology and Psychiatry*, 44, 489–508.

Murray, L. (1992). The impact of postnatal depression on infant development. *Journal of Child Psychology and Psychiatry*, 33, 534–561.

Murray, L., and Andrews, L. (2005). *The Social Baby*. (Richmond: The Children's Project)

Murray, L., Fiori-Cowley, A., Hooper, R., and Cooper, P.J. (1996). The impact of postnatal depression and associated adversity on early mother-infant interactions and later infant outcome. *Child Development*, 67, 2515–2526.

Murray, L., Woolgar, M., Cooper, P., and Hipwell, A. (2001). Cognitive vulnerability in five-year-old children of depressed mothers. *Journal of Child Psychology and Psychiatry*, 42, 891–899.

Panksepp, J., and Trevarthen, C. (2009). The neuroscience of emotion in music. In S. Malloch, and C. Trevarthen (eds) *Communicative Musicality*, pp. 105–146. (Oxford: OUP)

Papoušek, H. (1996). Musicality in infancy research: biological and cultural origins of early musicality. In I. Delige, and J. Sloboda (eds) *Musical Beginnings: Origins and Development of Musical Competence*, pp. 37–55. (New York: OUP)

Papoušek, M. (1996). Intuitive parenting: a hidden source of musical stimulation in infancy. In I. Delige, and J. Sloboda (eds) *Musical Beginnings: Origins and Development of Musical Competence*, pp. 88–112. (New York: OUP)

Pavlicevic, M. (1997). *Music Therapy in Context: Music, Meaning and Relationship* (London: Jessica Kingsley)

Perry, B., Pollard, R., Blakley, T., Baker, W., and Vigilante, D. (1995). Childhood trauma, the neurobiology of adaptation, and 'use-dependent' development of the brain: how states become traits. *Infant Mental Health Journal*, 16, 271–291.

Prior, V., and Glaser, D. (2006). *Understanding Attachment and Attachment Disorders* (London: Jessica Kingsley)

Robarts, J. (2009). Supporting the development of mindfulness and meaning: clinical pathways in music therapy with a sexually abused child. In S. Malloch, and C. Trevarthen (eds) *Communicative Musicality*, pp. 377–400. (Oxford: OUP)

Rustin, M. (1999). Multiple families in mind. *Clinical Child Psychology and Psychiatry*, 4, 51–62.

Salkeld, C. (2008). Music therapy after adoption: the role of family music therapy in developing secure attachment in adopted children. In A. Oldfield, and C. Flower (eds) *Music Therapy with Children and their Families*, pp. 141–158. (London: Jessica Kingsley)

Schore, A. (2001). The effects of early relational trauma on right-brain development, affect regulation, and infant mental health. *Infant Mental Health Journal*, 22, 201–269.

Stern, D. (1985). *The Interpersonal World of the Infant*. (New York: Basic Books)

Stewart, D. (1996). Chaos, noise and a wall of silence. *British Journal of Music Therapy*, 10, 21–33.

Trevarthen, C. (1979). Communication and cooperation in early infancy. A description of primary intersubjectivity. In M. Bullowa (ed.) *Before Speech: The Beginning of Human Communication*, pp. 321–347. (London: CUP)

Trevarthen, C. (1999). Musicality and the intrinsic motive pulse: evidence from human psychobiology and infant communication. *Musicae Scientiae*, Special Issue, 155–215.

Trevarthen, C., and Malloch, S. (2002). Musicality and music before three: human vitality and invention shared with pride. *Zero to Three*, 23, 10–18.

Wigram, T., and Elefant, C. (2009). Therapeutic dialogues in music: nurturing musicality of communication in children with autistic spectrum disorder and Rett syndrome. In S. Malloch, and C. Trevarthen (eds) *Communicative Musicality*, pp. 423–446. (Oxford: OUP)

Winnicott, D. (1990). *The Maturational Processes and the Facilitating Environment*. (London: Karnac Books)

Yule, W., Perrin, S., and Smith, P. (1999). Post-traumatic stress disorders in children and adolescents. In W. Yule (ed.) *Post Traumatic Stress Disorders*, pp. 25–50. (Chichester: John Wiley & Sons, Ltd)

Chapter 3

'The first time ever I saw your face . . .': Music therapy for depressed mothers and their infants

Alison Levinge

Four year old Daniel and his young mother have a difficult relationship and do not connect in a comfortable way. For Daniel's mother, the early years with her son had not been easy and as a result impacted upon her own feelings of self worth. In music therapy sessions we worked together to create a space in which successful relating could occur. As the musical relationship developed, Daniel began relating through his musical gestures which encouraged his mother to become more interactive. It would seem that by seeing her son play together with me in the music, she herself was brought to life.

Introduction

A baby's experiences take place in the context of a relationship. The quality and character of this first relationship are formed through the ways in which the baby and primary caregiver learn to be together, and are highly dependent upon a caregiver's availability. This availability is not about how much time can be spent with the baby literally. It is rather to do with the nature of the adult's presence, which as the paediatrician and psychoanalyst Donald Winnicott described, must be of the 'ordinary devoted' kind (Phillips 1988 p. 4).

The particular adult we eventually become, in part depends upon the kind of self which has formed and grown out of our early experience s of life. As adults, it is in the ways in which we manage different stresses and cope with the disruptions and unpredictable events which happen to us that we reveal something of how we were supported to do this when we were at our most vulnerable.

Through research arising from the establishment of a more 'complex psychoneurobiological model of the initial stages of the development of the mind, especially the unconscious mind' (Wilkinson 2006 p. vii) it is now possible to understand the impact our early experiences have upon our social development and ultimately upon the development of a self. From the combined areas of study in neurobiology and attachment theory, we now know that our early experiences of being with and being cared for by another are responsible for shaping the neural connections from which our minds ultimately develop (Siegel 1999). However, before considering the processes involved in developing a sense of self, I shall return to the music therapy clinical space where Daniel and his mother are searching for a way of being together.

Understanding Daniel and his mother

In this following example, we can see how music therapy is used to support the ability of the child to develop a greater repertoire of expression. Initially this will be with the therapist and then ultimately with the parent who will be supported to attend to her child differently and encouraged to initiate more rewarding exchanges. As these more positive connections become established they are able to carry into daily relating and can override the previous negative and unsuccessful failures of attempted intimacy.

In the clinical space I watch as mother and son take their places in the room away from each other. Mother sits perfectly still, as if not daring to move, whilst Daniel is sat on the floor playing on his own. He is deconstructing the xylophone, removing the bars one by one. As he does so, he talks to himself using a language only he can understand. I am seated at the piano. The counter transference feelings are powerful. In consequence, I find myself mirroring Daniel's mother's physical position in the way that I am seated, as well as expressing an aspect of the quality of helplessness in finding that I am unable to play the piano. I feel like a music mother who has slipped into a kind of coma. I am awake, yet trapped and I feel deskilled. As a group, it is as if we are three isolates, unable to play music and stuck in a state of unaliveness. After a while, his mother moves from her position seated across the room and places herself next to me. Daniel appears to ignore his mother's change of position and continues with his play. From the way he is behaving it would appear that he cannot believe there is a place for him in his mother's mind. Next Daniel picks up the beaters and hits the drum which prompts me to respond. In an attempt to make some small shift, I respond musically by playing a trill followed by a glissando on the piano. A look from Daniel toward me introduces an alive connection between us. Something in the way Daniel responds to my music, gives me the feeling that it is possible for a more sustained and lively connection to develop. Bringing the two beaters together, Daniel rubs them one upon the other. Perhaps this is a reflection of the way in which he and I have begun to form a musical connection. However, this moment is brief and he turns away moving toward the other side of the room. As he passes the glockenspiel, he accidentally knocks a few of the bars making a sound. This provides me with an opportunity for introducing a more sustained and melodic musical intervention. I play a melodically shaped musical phrase, which reflects and expands the qualities of this accidental music. This musical dialogue appears to release mother from her fixed position and she begins to become more visually engaged in what is happening. By continuing to play the piano, Daniel is physically brought back to the drum and psychically back to where he started near to mother and me. As the musical relationship develops Daniel appears to begin relating through his musical gestures, mother starts to become more involved. It would seem that by seeing her son play together with me in the music, she is brought to life herself.

My experience of this dyad in the music therapy sessions led me to believe that a positive sense of self had been difficult for Daniel to achieve. It seemed that his mother's own depressed feelings had prevented her from being totally available for her son and in consequence inhibited her capacity to provide Daniel with an alive and engaging presence. As the sessions continued, the musical aliveness became more present and robust and the relationship between Daniel and his mother began to flourish. Later in the therapeutic process mother and son came together literally, both in their musical exchanges and in the physicality of the ways in which their similar instruments, two horns, touched as they played. In this moment the music became a dialogue between mother and Daniel. As they connected I was able to take a third and more distant position and one in which I could support this couple musically from my place at the piano.

The developing infant: self and other

Different ways of understanding early development have established new insights and provided us with different ways of thinking about how the mind is, as Siegel (2003) points out '. . . shaped by the interaction of interpersonal experience and neurobiological processes.' As growth in this area is so dependent upon the quality of the first relationship, it has been understood that '. . . the kind of brain that each baby develops is the brain that comes out of his or her experiences with people.' (Gerhardt 2004 p. 38).The brain is 'experience dependent' (Gerhardt 2004 p. 38). From the very beginning of life the baby's brain develops in interaction with others, and as Siegel (2003) has described, a baby's early engagement with another 'shape the brain connections that create the mind and enable an emerging sense of "self" in the world' (Siegel 2003 p. 6).

The priority for a newborn baby is to be able to internally regulate his body systems. As Gerhardt tells us this is followed by the process of adaptation to external conditions. The baby learns to manage this mostly by using emotional responses and 'emotions are first and foremost our guides to self-regulation.' (Gerhardt 2004 p. 33). The development of the 'emotional brain' (p. 35) links to the development of the prefrontal cortex. This part of the brain[1] involves affect regulation needed for secure attachment (Fosha 2003) and links the sensory areas of the cortex with the emotional and survival-orientated subcortex. An important part of this area is known as the orbitofrontal cortex which develops after birth, and is 'so much about being human' (Gerhardt 2004 p. 37). It is this area which plays a key role in managing emotional life. As Schore has explained, 'attachment experiences, face to face transactions of affect synchrony between care-giver and infant, directly influence the imprinting, the circuit wiring of the orbitofrontal cortex . . .' (Schore 2003 p. 60).

The amygdala is the part of the brain responsible for processing the infant's responses to its caregiver. In particular, the amygdala involves processing the emotional expressions of the face (Sieratzki and Woll 1996). As a protection it organizes a brain–body response. It is the role of the cortex to moderate the response of the amygdala. However, if the baby does not experience enough positive social interactions, then the capacity of the cortex to override this primitive response may not develop sufficiently. It is also here in the amygdala that memories of an unconscious nature are stored and 'form the early patterning that dictates the most deeply held ways of being and behaving that become part of our emotional repertoire for the rest of our lives' (Wilkinson 2006 p. 25).

Psychological and neurological research has demonstrated that a developing self requires certain conditions. These conditions are created by the ways in which a mother or primary caregiver relates to her baby and are developed through the way she attunes to her baby's different states of being. Winnicott (1952) believed that in the beginning, a baby's self is an 'inherited potential' (Winnicott 1952 p. 99) which can only develop if linked to quality maternal care. He proposed that 'There is no such thing as a baby' and explained that '. . . if you show me a baby you certainly show me also someone caring for the baby,

---

[1] This is the part of the brain at the back of the frontal lobes. It is implicated in functions such as moderation of social behaviours, planning and carrying out complex cognitive tasks, and the development of personality.

or at least a pram with someone's eyes and ears glued to it. One sees a "nursing couple"' (Winnicott 1952: p. 99).

Winnicott maintained that an infant's development could not be separated from the quality of care it receives and that these two elements are intertwined. His lifetime of observation and study of families, led him to state that it is a mother, or primary caregiver, along with the quality of caring interactions which '*makes* the *becoming* self of the infant feasible.' (Khan 1992 p. xxxvii). Winnicott considered that it is a mother's ability to attune to her baby which helps to provide the 'good enough' conditions in which her baby can develop. The particular kind of attunement required is one which connects with what the baby is feeling as well as to what the baby is doing. This capacity for attunement arises out of a mother's gradual acknowledgement of her infant's spontaneous gestures, in what ever form or shape they appear. Initially a baby's sense of self is placed in the body. Therefore what we learn about the world at the beginning of life, is held not just in what Wilkinson names as our 'mind brain' (Wilkinson 2006 p. 16), but also in our body.

Initially, one of the strongest means by which attachment takes place is through visual contact accompanied by vocal sounds. The mother's expressions and responses to her baby's gestures, enables her baby to experience himself as being 'seen for what he in fact (is)' and more significantly '. . . at any moment' (Phillips 1988 p. 130). Winnicott described this process in what could be described as being like a short poem:

> When I look I am seen, so I exist.
> I can now afford to look and see.
> I now look creatively and what I apperceive I also perceive.
> In fact I take care not to see what is not there to be seen (unless I am tired).
>
> (Winnicott 1971 p. 154)

'Not to be seen by the mother, at least at the moment of the spontaneous gesture, is not to exist.' (Phillips 1988 p. 130). So if a baby is forced to read their caregiver's moods at their own expense, then the developing sense of self may become compromised. This way of looking provided by the mother at first provides instant images which are invested with emotion. Later these become 'lasting images . . . images of self with another . . . but etched in memory' (Gerhardt 2004 p. 47). This positive gaze between the caregiver and infant is a vital stimulus to the growth of what has been described as the 'social brain' (Gerhardt 2004 p. 35).

Other ways of identifying with her baby come through her acknowledgement of the infant's gestures, whether these are movements, expressions, or sounds, a parent can begin to identify with the baby. This becomes a kind of dance, the impact of which is to create a to-and-fro process of communication, which in turn contributes to forming a 'psychological bond' (Decety and Chaminade 2003 p. 579). Humans learn not just from the other but also through the other. Therefore the ways in which a mother holds, handles and manages her baby contributes to what the baby will eventually internalize about how themselves. These experiences will contribute towards building an internal representation of what it means to be with another person. As Gerhardt wrote, 'Our minds emerge and our emotions become organised through engagement with other minds, not in isolation' (Gerhardt 2004 p. 15).

Winnicott proposed that the availability of a 'good enough' mother was necessary for the infant's psychological survival and development. This means that the caregiver has to be able to have a space in her mind where she can symbolically hold her baby and consider all of the baby's needs. This is not the kind of thinking which is mechanical, but one which shapes the baby's emotional responses to life. The mind enables us to process information and regulate how we adapt to the environment. In other words, 'the mind can alter the brain and the brain can alter the mind' (Siegel 2003 p. 9). Therefore, as part of her capacity to think, a mother who can help to moderate the experiences of her infant enables a thinking rather than a reacting mind to develop in her infant, and she facilitates the processes which go toward allowing her baby to develop his or her own mechanisms for self-regulation.

Problems in relating and their consequences

In Bernard MacLaverty's novel *Grace Notes*, a fictional mother is described as becoming overwhelmed by her feelings of depression. In this narrative she appears tortured by her baby as the grind of the daily routine obliterates the brightness of her days, forming a darkness which descends upon her 'step by step' (MacLaverty 1998 p. 201). This ever increasing gloom incapacitates her, affecting her state of mind and disabling her ability to empathize with her baby. Described in vivid and raw terms, the mother of this novel finds herself feeling lonely and isolated, and unable to bear the inevitable neediness her baby evokes in her.

This story of a struggling new mother poignantly describes the kind of feelings someone suffering from post-natal depression may have. The symptoms experienced can be so incapacitating as to make it difficult to seek help. Locked in a frightening and disabling state of mind, a mother's feelings may be complex. Her feelings of vulnerability may evoke a wish to be looked after and this may be expressed through a desire to be hospitalized for example. She may even find herself hoping that her baby might not wake up. These feelings are disturbing, frightening, and difficult to bear, and as in the case of the mother depicted in the novel, impact on how a mother will relate to her baby.

Part of a mother or primary caregiver's role is to help the baby to develop a capacity for managing stress. By presenting life in manageable doses, the infant is helped not to become overwhelmed. This particular function of mothering provides what has been named a 'protective shield' (Khan 1986 p. 46). Through the availability of the caregiver for providing this function on behalf of the infant and at a time when the infant cannot manage this themselves, the infant can be helped to increasingly self-regulate the feelings which arise from daily life events. If the baby is not helped to manage the stresses which naturally arise, and these stresses continue, then this may ultimately inhibit the development of a strong enough bond between caregiver and baby. The baby is then vulnerable to ongoing stress through not having developed adequate regulatory mechanisms.

> Prolonged and frequent episodes of intense and unregulated stress in infants and toddlers has devastating effects on the establishment of psychophysiological regulation and upon the development of stable and trusting attachment relationships in the first year of life.
>
> (Gaensbauer and Siegel 1995 p. 294)

Maternal depression

When a mother is depressed, and particularly if the depression is severe, then this can interfere with her ability to tune into her infant's signals and in consequence may inhibit her capacity to provide the sensitive and emotionally nurturing environment the infant requires. This inability to be available to her baby in the way he or she needs can result in insecure attachment which has lifelong consequences for enjoying life and coping with adversity (Campbell et al. 2004). As Gerhardt (2004 p. 123) has described, when children of depressed parents grow up they are at about six times greater risk of succumbing to depression themselves. Babies of depressed mothers may avoid making eye contact and even become withdrawn.

A mother with post-natal depression can express the feelings which arise from this mood disorder in different ways. For example, she may appear disconnected and absent from her infant, or in contrast, may be over active and behave intrusively toward her infant. Some mothers, who are experiencing severe depression, may even find it difficult to believe that their infant is really theirs.

These different behaviours have been seen to appear in the case of the withdrawn state, 40 per cent of the time (Gerhardt 2004). In this state mothers who are depressed can be seen to be unresponsive or disengaged '. . . whilst much of the rest of the time she will be angry, intrusive and rough with their babies' (Gerhardt 2004 p. 124). In response to this kind of care, these babies look away from their mothers a lot. In turn, this can evoke more intrusive and demanding behaviours from their mothers. As depressed mothers can find it difficult to respond to their babies and tend to be apathetic and withdrawn, their babies may therefore experience 'more negative than positive feelings' (Gerhardt 2004 p. 124). In contrast to the more absent quality of a mother's presence, a mother who behaves intrusively and in a covertly angry way reveals her depression through the ways in which she handles her infant. For example, she may pick the infant up in an aggressive manner, or act abruptly when interacting. In response the infant may become insecurely attached in a disorganized way (Main and Soloman 1986).

Therapeutic work with depressed mothers and their infants

As a therapeutic process which is inherently interactive, music therapy can provide an effective means by which difficult relationships between a mother and her baby can be helped to change. The problems which can be observed in therapy with young children usually have begun at an earlier stage of development when a baby is starting to form a sense of self. At this time, the infant is at his or her most vulnerable and totally dependent upon his or her mother for physical and psychological needs. The work of therapy with depressed mothers and their infants is to ameliorate these established difficulties through exploring new ways of relating.

When early attachment issues are a concern, and when possible, therapy should be carried out with the mother and her child together. It is important not to see the difficulties as residing with either the mother or the infant alone, but to understand the child and parent as a system and be prepared to work with both members of the dyad together.

As a music therapist and according to their needs, I use different ways of working therapeutically with mothers and their infants. One way is to work with the dyad alone, as described in the example of Daniel and his mother. In this work, I use direct and specifically tailored musical interventions appropriate to the mother and child's needs, and these will be carried out in a predominantly non-directive way and taking the lead from whatever the mother and child are doing or how they are being. Another way of working is in a group format, where several dyads come together and the group works as a unit facilitated by a music therapist and co-therapist where possible. Each way of working brings its own particular dynamics which must be included in consideration of the meaning of the interactions in the therapeutic work.

When working in a group of mothers and their babies, a number of different dynamic levels are evoked. Therefore the intensity of the work is expanded and amplified and interactions between all the members happen at a number of different levels. These include: (a) the dyad itself, mother to infant and infant to mother; (b) a mother's relationship to the music therapist; (c) a mother's relationship to other mothers; (d) an infant's relationship to other babies/mothers; and (e) each infant's/mother's relationship toward the musical interventions.

Assessment of needs

Referrals are received through various professional channels according to the setting in which the work is carried out. In my case, being part of a service offered to Children Centres, children and their mothers are referred usually by health visitors, or other professionals connected to family services.

When a mother is finding it difficult to be with her child in a satisfying way then often she will experience negative feelings about herself and her ability to mother her infant. Therefore it will be necessary to find a way of getting alongside her in order that she can feel comfortable before beginning the work. This can be done through visiting the home, preferably with someone already known to the mother, such as the health visitor.

Once a connection is established, an assessment will be carried out. If a mother has been diagnosed with depression then it is likely that a medical assessment will already have been conducted. For the purposes of music therapy however, I carry out an assessment of needs which also includes taking a family history and is an essential part of the mother–child work that I provide. As there is increasing evidence that there is an association between 'the way in which a mother recalls her own childhood experience and the quality of the relationship existing between her and her child' (Fonagy et al. 1991 p. 891) it is important to ascertain as much information as is possible about all family relationships. Babies can become the carriers of a mother's unconscious fears and difficulties so it is important, through discussion, to find out how a mother views her child and to try to understand how she sees their relationship. When possible, and this may come later in the work, helping a mother to express some of her own feelings about being mothered, will support the work and as her understanding of herself develops, enable some differentiation to develop between her own experiences as a child and her current role as a mother.

The therapeutic role of the music therapist

In the therapeutic work it can be more helpful to a mother or caregiver if the therapist is able to stand back, and take the position of someone who is at more of a psychological and emotional distance, as if representing a third generation.

From this place, the therapist can be used positively to help a mother become more aware of her own capacity for being good enough. As music mothers or even music grandmothers, the most significant elements of our role therefore, is to affirm a mother's capacity for mothering and to carry on their behalf, the projections which arise from the work. In other words, in order to support change, as music therapists we need not only to feel but also contain what the mothers themselves are feeling. As therapy will inevitably connect to primitive feelings expressed within the mother–baby relationship, this can be difficult and at times painful. As therapists however, we are there to be a witness to the pain of our clients and not to avoid it.

As in any group process, in the beginning the members will look toward the facilitator for guidance and support. As music therapists we are not exempt from this dynamic. Equally our musical expertise provides us with another attribute which can be admired, feared or envied by those in the group. In working with mothers, caregivers and their babies the kind of projective identification associated with being seen as the 'expert' can mean that as therapists we can easily be thought of as being a 'better mother' and one with 'all the goodies'. If this is not sensitively managed, our role in the group may only confirm a mother's already low self esteem and in consequence add to her feelings about not being a 'good enough' mother to her baby. For example, as in the time when a mother commented to me as I sang along with a group that she felt that her son had listened to my voice rather than to hers. In that moment as I connected vocally, the relating couple became me and the baby, leaving the natural mother to feel left out and striving to establish her place.

It is possible that witnessing the struggles of a depressed mother in relating to her baby may drive a therapist toward intervening and in consequence, can evoke competitive behaviour with the mother. These experiences are easily evoked when the mothers themselves are feeling so depleted, and by comparison as therapists we can appear so rich in resources. It can be difficult to stand back and support the mother and infant to find their way together. However, this is required of a therapist in order to create spaces available for ongoing work. Professional development, supervision, and the self-reflection of the therapist are therefore essential to being able to work effectively.

When the American psychoanalyst Beatrice Beebe was videotaped working with babies in despair, she reported that 'in order not to fail the infant, she had to sit and do nothing, just to be with the infant and not to encourage her to be other than she was, in despair' (Davis 1999 p. 267). By attuning to the actual feelings of the infant, the infant can feel 'met' and become hopeful again.

The music in music therapy

Music is by its nature interactive. Therefore, in a therapeutic context it can provide a means by which a therapist can literally tune into the 'here and now' elements of a relationship. This is particularly relevant for a mother and her baby, as in the early stages of development the baby is building a picture of itself moment by moment.

Unlike the therapeutic work with individual dyads, working in a group of couples requires some structure. This is in order that the varied complex feelings arising from the number of mothers and their babies taking part may be contained and a space for play created. In my own clinical work this structure has been developed initially through the use of pre-composed songs, based upon tunes which are familiar to the mothers, such as nursery rhymes. Words which are relevant to the aims of the group replace the original text, grounding the music in the therapeutic work.

For example, references to body parts supported by actions can encourage a mother to touch and physically connect with her baby's bodily self. Songs based on making visual connections enable a mother to focus upon the facial expressions of her baby and strengthen the process of attunement. So, singing her baby's name whilst making eye contact can help to support development of this connection further by creating a stronger sense of identification. Considering the actual individual elements of music, each one can be used in specific ways to support a mother becoming more sensitive to her baby's needs. For example, rhythmic emphasis within the context of a tempo tailored to the group's sense of timing, can enable a mother to handle her baby in a more sensitive way and help her learn how to literally time her responses so that they meet her baby's physical expressions and movements.

Using her voice, which is at the centre of most of the musical interventions, helps a mother to develop a natural means of making connections with her baby. Being depressed can inhibit a mother's ability to vary the pitch, tone and quality of her vocalizations. Singing in a group can support a mother in finding her own authentic voice and enable her to become more expressive and therefore more available to her baby.

One of the most meaningful therapeutic interventions of the work is clinical improvisation. During this time, neither any musical direction nor specific time boundary is suggested. Mothers and their babies are encouraged to play as freely as they wish and in whatever way they wish. In my experience, it is during this particular musical intervention supported by the increasing familiarity with the environment, that the feeling element of each relationship becomes vividly present. More spontaneous and sensitive connections and responses can be seen between mothers and their babies and as the group becomes more relaxed, different musical ideas are developed and tried.

Group music therapy for depressed mothers and their infants

Two examples of work in a group follow, illustrating some of the difficulties a mother and her baby may experience whilst trying to engage.

Julie brings her son into the clinical space and lays him down on the cushion provided. She remains standing whilst Harvey lies still and almost lifeless. The group starts and we are all singing a 'Hello' song. The mothers are asked to sing first to the group members and then to their baby. Julie tries to engage Harvey as she sings his name, but he turns away, first toward one side then the other, each time avoiding mother's gaze. Becoming desperate, mother leans further in toward Harvey almost touching his face with hers. Still he does not look, but instead arches his back pulling further away from his mother. Finally, and appearing to give up, mother turns her son around to face the group.

Whilst this is only a moment in one of the sessions, observation suggests that this is an avoidantly attached dyad. The mother has had to work very hard to engage her baby, resulting in her exhibiting what has been described as 'looming behaviour' (Beebe and Lachmann 2002 p. 37). This means that in order to connect with her baby, a mother has to lean over her baby in order to chase the contact that the baby is trying to avoid. Here, Harvey could not escape the face of his mother and as a result the arching of his body gave expression to his anxious feelings of this experience. It may be that Harvey will have internalized the feelings created by this encounter and in consequence find difficulty in developing a positive connection with his mother.

As described previously, depression presents itself in different ways. Sometimes a mother may be absent and distant from her baby like the mother of Harvey. Alternatively, a mother's depression may lead her to feel that she has to be seen to be actively connecting with her baby and consequently intervene in ways which do not allow her baby the right kind of time to process the connections. In this next example we see how this mother finds difficulty in waiting for her baby to respond.

Margaret sits her baby down on the cushion and kneels in front of him in readiness for the improvisation. Unable to wait for her baby to play the instrument he is holding, Margaret intervenes grabbing the maraca whilst held in her baby's hand and shaking it. In response her baby becomes frustrated and begins to cry. This crying is too much for Margaret to bear and as a way of managing the feelings evoked, she quickly changes the instrument for something different. Her baby looks momentarily stunned as events move faster than he is able to process.

In Margaret's attempts to help her baby join the activities of the group as described above, I found that I was prompted to intervene. For the sake of this mother's capacity for mothering to develop, it was essential that my own feelings be contained, as this could have been experienced as a repeat or mirroring of the previous intrusive behaviour carried out by the mother toward her baby. Instead, the co-therapist in the group moved over to sit by Margaret and her baby, and in order to provide some holding gently played alongside. It was hoped that by supporting this mother, and not responding to the counter transference feelings evoked, she could then allow her baby the time he needed to be able to play in his own way.

As the sessions continued, the mothers and caregivers appeared to be more comfortable both in their ability to express themselves musically, as well as in their interactions and interventions with their babies. This is seen particularly in the clinical improvisation element of the music making. Each week the length of time for free improvisation naturally increased and the mothers and caregivers were able to be more playful and spontaneous with their babies. As a result, the interactions are more creative and the expressions and responses more alive and meaningful between them. In this final example we see how mother and baby were able to play creatively as the mother's ability to be present increased.

In the penultimate session Sarah and her baby are rolling the bell backwards and forwards between them. This to-and-fro movement made in time to one of the songs is carried out in an atmosphere of calm and playfulness. Mother looks directly at her baby Lisa as the game continues and the positive visual connection is clearly helping to cement their relationship. At one point, seated near her mother, Lisa jumps up and down in time to the music, a movement which mother spontaneously mirrors with her own body both in time and shape.

As a mother's depression begins to lift she is able to be more alive in responding to her baby's expressions and gestures. The couple in this example show they have found a way of being together in a more satisfying and creative way and as mother's depression begins to lift she is able to be more alive in responding to her baby's expression and gestures.

Summary and conclusion

The natural interactive element of music provides mothers who are depressed with a non-verbal means by which they may connect with their baby. Equally, the temporal nature of music, allows for sensitive and empathic attunement to be developed in the moment between therapist and mother, therapist and child, and mother and child.

Musical communication involves the use of touch, sight and hearing. Using music in therapeutic work, we can elaborate and amplify what is happening in any one moment, thus supporting positive and sensitive interpersonal communications. Positive and negative affect can be experienced by the baby or child through such means as the melodic shape of the mother's sounds, the speed or timing of her delivery or through her facial and bodily expressions. Musical play allows these expressions to be practised, repeated and enjoyed following a supportive musical structure provided by the therapist and experienced between the mother and her infant.

The therapeutic use of music can meet, match and support both the non-verbal as well as verbal ways in which a mother relates, whilst at the same time as holding the different complex feelings which arise within the musical container created by the therapist. In a music therapy relationship, it is easy to see how a baby and mother can be engaged on a visual, vocal and physical level as they play with the instruments. However, more importantly, music can reflect the feeling element of the sound gestures, and find a connection with all the various ways in which the expressions and different communications are made between a mother and her baby. This may have been unsuccessfully attempted by the mother in play at home, or not attempted at all. In providing the right environment for this interplay to be nurtured, the music therapist supports the development of essential skills in the mother, with ongoing benefits to the dyad.

One of the most significant musical ways of interaction a mother has is her voice. Once born, a baby naturally seeks to bond with his or her mother. However, whilst still in the womb a baby makes a connection to his or her mother through recognition of her voice. This connection is made even before the baby enters the world. Once in the world, the pitch of a mother's vocal expressions conveys not only the quality of her actual vocal sounds, but also the meaning or intention behind her expressions and actions. Gradually her baby learns to understand the meaning of these sounds.

For a mother who finds relating to her baby difficult, the therapeutic use of music can provide a means by which significant steps may be taken to transform disconnections into connections. The intensity of music therapy work with mothers, caregivers and their children, particularly in a group, means that there is much to observe. The more intense the dynamics, the more need there is for understanding the details of these processes. The primary aim of work with a child and his or her mother or caregiver, as a couple or within a group setting, is to strengthen the attachment.

A mother who is depressed and therefore limited in her ability to be available for her infant will take time to be helped. An infant does not have that time.

An infant needs to be supported in developing social and emotional competence. Given that an infant and mother form a relational system in themselves, then it follows that enabling change in one partner to happen may influence change in the other.

Change in therapy between mothers and infants occurs when there has been a special moment of attunement. Music therapy is used both to support and create these moments encouraging mothers and caregivers to be more attuned to their child's expressions and gestures and as a result, develop a stronger attachment. The earlier that therapeutic work can happen, the more likely later difficulties can be prevented. As Balbernie, a child and family service practitioner wrote: 'The time of greatest influence, for good or ill, is when the brain is new. If we want to help the next generation we should be working with their parents while they are babies now' (Balbernie 2001 p. 253).

References

Balbernie, R. (2001). Circuits and circumstances: the neurobiological consequences of early relationship experiences and how they shape behaviour. *Journal of Child Psychotherapy*, 27, 237–255.

Beebe, B., and Lachmann, F.M. (2002). *Infant Research and Adult Treatment*. (Hillsdale, NJ: The Analytic Press)

Campbell, S.B., Brownell, C.A., Hungerford, A., Spieker, S., Mohan, R., and Blessing, J.S. (2004). The course of maternal depressive symptoms and maternal sensitivity as predictors of preschool attachment security at 36 months. *Development and Psychopathology*, 16, 231–252.

Davis, M. (1999). Mind, body, or self: the analysis of a 16 year old girl with hysterical psychosis. *Association for Child Psychoanalysis Newsletter*, 9–10.

Decety, J., and Chaminade, T. (2003). When the self represents the other: a new cognitive neuroscience view on psychological identification. *Consciousness and Cognition*, 12, 577–596.

Fonagy, P., Steele, H., and Steele, M. (1991). Maternal representations of attachment during pregnancy predict the organization of infant-mother attachment at one year of age. *Child Development*, 62, 891–905.

Fosha, D. (2003). Dyadic regulation and experiential work with emotion and relatedness in trauma and disordered attachment. In D.J. Siegel and M.F. Solomon (eds) *Healing Trauma: Attachment, Trauma, the Brain and the Mind*, pp. 221–281. (New York: Norton)

Gaensbauer, T., and Siegel, C.H. (1995). Therapeutic approaches to posttraumatic stress disorder in infants and toddlers. *Infant Mental Health Journal*, 16, 292–305.

Gerhardt, S. (2004). *Why Love Matters: How Affection Shapes a Baby's Brain*. (New York; Brunner-Routledge)

Khan, M. (1986). *The Privacy of the Self*. (London: The Hogarth Press and The Institute of Psycho-Analysis)

Khan, M. (1992). Introduction. In D.W. Winnicott *Through Paediatrics to Psycho-Analysis*, p. xxxvii. (London: Karnac Books)

MacLaverty, B. (1998). *Grace Notes: a Novel*. (London: Norton)

Main, M., and Solomon J. (1986). Discovery of an insecure-disorganized/disoriented attachment pattern. In T.B. Brazelton and M.W. Yogman (eds) *Affective Development in Infancy*, pp. 95–124. (Norwood, NJ: Ablex)

Phillips, A. (1988). *Winnicott.* (London: Fontana)

Schore, A.N. (2003). *Affect Dysregulation and Repair of the Self.* (New York: Norton)

Siegel, D. (1999). *The Developing Mind: Toward a Neurobiology of Interpersonal Experience.* (New York: Guilford)

Siegel, D.J. (2003). An interpersonal neurobiology of psychotherapy: the developing mind and the resolution of trauma. In M. Solomon, and D.J. Siegel (eds) *Healing Trauma: Attachment, Trauma, the Brain and the Mind*, pp.1–56. (New York: Norton)

Sieratzki, J.S., and Woll, B. (1996). Why do mothers cradle babies on their left? *Lancet*, 347, 1746–1748.

Wilkinson, M. (2006). *Coming into Mind: the Mind-Brain Relationship: a Jungian Clinical Perspective.* (London: Routledge)

Winnicott, D.W. (1952). *Through Paediatrics to Psychoanalysis: Collected Papers.* (London: Karnac)

Winnicott, D.W. (1971). *Playing and Reality.* (London: Tavistock)

Chapter 4

Parents' perceptions of being in music therapy sessions with their children: What is our role as music therapists with parents?

Amelia Oldfield

From the very beginning, Sam has been happy to attend music therapy. Initially, he found it very difficult to wait for the sessions to start. I tried to time our arrival at the Child Development Centre so that we didn't get there too early – waiting around was very difficult at that time for Sam. He would run around the waiting room and climb on chairs, etc. However, once we sat down in Amelia's room and she started to play the guitar and sing the 'Hello' song, he would become very calm. He would sit down on his chair. He made good eye contact with Amelia, smiling at her as she sang to him. He would strum or tap on the guitar when it was offered to him and join in with the music making. But it was the absolute look of delight on his face when Amelia was singing to him that completely convinced me that he was happy to be there and really engaged. He was also happy for me to be part of the sessions.

Sam's mother, Laura

Introduction

For the past 11 years, parents of individual pre-school children I have seen at the Child Development Centre, Addenbrookes, Cambridge, have been actively involved in their children's music therapy sessions. I am convinced that it is essential to include parents in these sessions and I have published articles and chapters about the importance of parents being in the sessions (Oldfield 2001, 2006a, 2008). Seven parents I have worked with have written positively about the experience of being in music therapy sessions (Oldfield 2006a, 2008). In my PhD research investigation (Oldfield 2004) 10 parents were interviewed who reported favourably about the music therapy processes in which they had been involved.

As I have written elsewhere, I have become so used to working with parents in the room that 'One part of my brain is automatically focused on the parent and the parent's needs . . .' (Oldfield 2008 p. 20). However, when looking at my written music therapy reports about individual children and their parents, it is interesting to note that the bulk of the report is about the child with only a sentence or two about the parent's involvement. Somehow, in these written reports it is easier and perhaps 'safer' to focus on the progress that the child has made. The work that has occurred with the parent is equally important but not always so clearly defined and often more difficult to bring out into the open.

In this chapter I consider the role of the music therapist with parents by focusing on the following topics: (a) original reasons for coming to music therapy; (b) initial uncertainty; (c) rejoicing in their child's enjoyment of the music; (d) non-verbal interactions; (e) containing and addressing difficult behaviours; and (f) working in partnership with parents.

I look specifically at parents' perceptions of being in music therapy sessions with their children and try to determine what our role as music therapists is with parents who are in the room with us. Laura's written account of 10 months of weekly music therapy sessions with her son, Sam, opens this investigation. All the children I refer to are between the ages of 2 and 4 and have communication difficulties. Most of the children have a diagnosis of autistic spectrum disorder. All the children described here happen to be boys, but I do also work with girls.

Sam and Laura

I worked with Sam and Laura for 9 months between September and July, seeing them for 30 minute weekly sessions at the Child Development Centre, Addenbrookes, during term time. I asked Laura to write about her perception of our work together. She wrote a first draft and then added a few paragraphs after seeing the book about music therapy with children and families which was published in May 2008 (Oldfield and Flower 2008).

This was what Laura wrote:

Sam was diagnosed with an autistic spectrum disorder when he was 2 years and 10 months old. By the time we received the official diagnosis, we were pretty sure that Sam had autism. His speech was very delayed and the words that he did use were lifted from films or books. He really didn't appear to have any understanding of the language that he was using or hearing others use. He was very active–he really couldn't sit still. I believe he was very frustrated by his lack of ability to communicate and also his lack of understanding of what was expected of him. He would lash out and become aggressive if someone was trying to stop him doing something. He would pull me around by the hand to try and show me what he wanted and, as it was sometimes impossible to work out what he was trying to show or tell me, he would become very frustrated. Looking back, I think that from about the age of 2½ (when his autistic tendencies became more apparent), he was a very frustrated and sometimes unhappy little boy.

I had taken Sam to music groups since he was a very little baby. He has always enjoyed music. He is alert, interested and engaged around music in a way that he often doesn't appear to be in other 'play' situations. He has also always been more inclined to cooperate with a request if it is sung to him, for example 'This is the way we put on our shoes' to the tune of the 'Mulberry Bush'. From a very young age, I took Sam to a music group in our village which Sam enjoyed. However, he did find it difficult sometimes if the group was large. He didn't like to sit but would run around the room and sometimes hide under a table if it became very noisy.

After Sam's diagnosis, I asked the Clinical Psychologist at the Child Development Centre in Cambridge if we could be referred for music therapy. I had heard that it might be available and I believed that Sam would benefit from it, although I wasn't really sure what the format of the sessions would be. A few months later, we were invited in for an assessment session with Amelia Oldfield. The first session we attended seemed to go well, although Sam wasn't terribly cooperative. He didn't appear to be anxious in the new surroundings and was happy to join in with some of the music making. We were offered the opportunity to attend regular music therapy sessions soon after this.

From the very beginning, Sam has been happy to attend music therapy. Initially, he found it very difficult to wait for the sessions to start. I tried to time our arrival at the Child Development Centre so that we didn't get there too early–waiting around was very difficult at that time for Sam. He would run around the waiting room and climb on chairs, etc. However, once we sat down in Amelia's room and she started to play the guitar and sing the 'Hello' song, he would become very calm. He would sit down on his chair. He made good eye contact with Amelia, smiling at her as she sang to him. He would strum or tap on the guitar when it was offered to him and join in with the music making. But it was the absolute look of delight on his face when Amelia was singing to him that completely convinced me that he was happy to be there and really engaged. He was also happy for me to be part of the sessions.

During the sessions, Sam is offered lots of choices of different instruments. Initially, he didn't manage very well making choices. As time has gone on, he has become much more willing to choose different instruments rather than repetitively going through the same routine each week. He enjoys playing the drums. He sometimes plays very loudly–almost aggressively– but his energy is channelled towards the drums and does not spill over into the session.

It's almost as if he is getting it all out of his system. At other times, he likes to play with the egg shakers by arranging them into very precise star shapes and patterns on the floor. He is given a little time to play and arrange the shapes as he wants but then he is redirected to another activity with the instruments.

Amelia has consistently used the same phrase '1, 2, 3 . . . finished' to indicate the end of an activity and Sam has accepted this and, from very early on in the sessions, has joined in with the counting down. This is something that I've taken away from music and we use at home as it can be very difficult to move Sam on from one activity to another and he absolutely recognizes this phrase as meaning something is 'finished'.

As the sessions have progressed, Sam has started to use more and more language, which is very exciting. Not just to indicate what he doesn't want, but also to suggest songs, instruments and develop games that Amelia instigates. This is an enormous step forward for Sam as, instead of wanting the session to be all on his terms, he's becoming happier with letting someone else take the lead and direct him. I find this very exciting because Sam will, to some extent, take direction from me but to see him now listening and following instructions from someone else is such a huge step forward. He does seem to be paying much more attention to what Amelia wants him to do. He's not always cooperative but he is increasingly responding to her direction in a positive way.

However, there have been times when his attention and cooperation have wavered. Shortly before the Easter holidays, he became less involved. He seemed to lose interest in some of the activities. He would roll around on the floor and refuse to participate. He would hide behind a screen or get caught up in repetitive activities or acting out scenes from films or books. It was difficult to keep him engaged and he seemed less interested and cooperative. I found this frustrating because music therapy had always been such a positive activity. Music generally had always been a very effective way of communicating with Sam and I really didn't want to lose this. Amelia and I discussed the changes and she suggested that maybe he had become a little bored with the routine of the sessions. Interestingly, at that time, Sam was being rather difficult in other areas. Amelia introduced a number of different instruments, games and activities. She has also always allowed Sam to have some control over what happens in the sessions. I have never felt that Amelia expects total compliance from Sam. Every little achievement that he makes in the sessions is celebrated.

From the beginning, I was unsure what my role would be in the sessions. I suppose I thought I was there to accompany Sam. I wasn't sure that I would be joining in with the music making. However, I do and I am glad that I can. Although I participate in the sessions, Amelia leads them and I am able to observe him playing/working with someone else. This has been very rewarding. His use of appropriate language has really improved, although he does sometimes need someone who is familiar with his speech to 'interpret' and I am glad to be able to do that as it helps to avoid frustration. His ability and willingness to make choices has also developed. This has been something that has been very difficult for Sam in the past and it helps him to communicate what he does and doesn't want. When he does get caught in a repetitive activity or speech loop, it is easier to distract him and redirect him. He is learning that he doesn't have to control every activity. He quite often still wants a song of his choice and in the past he would have objected to anyone else trying to join in and sing along. Now, he lets Amelia play along to his songs at the piano. In the past, if he had had enough of an activity, he would indicate the end. Now, he is more willing to allow the activity to carry on until Amelia agrees it's time to finish. The important thing for me is that he is willing to participate on someone else's terms. Were I not able to attend the sessions, I would not know how much he enjoys them and how well he participates. Being there, in the sessions, I can see that he loves to play the 'rainbow bells' and the xylophones–he could never explain that to me. It may seem a little selfish, but I don't want to miss out on those special activities. It also gives me ideas for activities we can try at home.

I believed that music therapy would be good for Sam as he has always enjoyed music, songs, rhythms, etc. (His ability to copy rhythms that Amelia beats out on the drum machine is fabulous and he is so pleased with himself when he gets it right.) What has been particularly exciting is seeing how it isn't just about the music. He has learned to share, to take turns (which he really finds very difficult in so many situations), to participate on someone else's terms. He seems happy to have a go at new activities during the sessions rather than sticking to the same safe activities week after week.

I hope that Sam will continue to enjoy music. He will receive music therapy at school, although I will not attend those sessions. Amelia has taught Sam a couple of short phrases from songs on the piano. He recently treated the family to a recital of 'Three Blind Mice' on the piano at home. There was much cheering and clapping and his little face just beamed with pride. I would like Sam to have more formal music tuition in the future. I think that it would be a great confidence booster for him to continue to develop this particular interest. He still is delighted every week when Amelia sings the 'Hello' song. Now at the end of the session, he wants us all to join in playing on the bongo drums for the 'Goodbye' song.

A music therapist's perception of the sessions

I have included almost all of the account written by Laura so that a full picture of her perception of the sessions is available. Much of what I might write about the work overlaps with what Laura has written so I will now just add a few thoughts of my own before reflecting on Laura and other parents' perceptions of being part of music therapy sessions.

Every week I particularly look forward to working with Sam and Laura. Sam is not only enthusiastic, lively and engaged, but also very creative, both musically and visually. He makes up beautiful star shapes with the instruments on the mat and then allows me to sing about them, picking up on my vocal intonation and my rhythmic patterns. His musical and artistic suggestions inspire me to improvise and respond, and the music between the three of us often flows easily and spontaneously.

As Laura has indicated, we have used the sessions to work on a number of non-musical objectives such as: (a) giving Sam an opportunity to express himself through music making; (b) helping Sam to develop his vocalizations and speech; and (c) helping Sam to accept direction and compromise. Over the past 9 months he has made great progress in all these areas. He will often play the drums or the piano extremely loudly and energetically, and appears to release some energy through this process. However, in between this forceful and sometimes aggressive playing, Sam will suddenly play very quietly, grinning widely at his musical joke and delighting in my expected and sometimes unexpected musical responses.

Sam's language has greatly improved. He will now echo back long sentences such as 'this is Sam's way of playing the drum' which we accompany with rhythmic patterns on the drum machine. He will also now use two- or three-word sentences to indicate what he wants, for example, 'more xylophone' or 'finish on the piano'.

As Sam has been able to trust me and the familiar structure of the session, he has been able to accept my choices and suggestions as well as enjoying familiar responses by myself and Laura to his chosen instruments and activities. In the last few weeks he has allowed me to show him the first few notes of 'Three Blind Mice' although it was essential that there was an element of free noisy improvisation during the longer phrase: 'They all ran after the farmer's wife, who . . .'. The free playing would maintain his interest until the end of the song, when he could finish with the three notes he knew for 'Three Blind Mice'. At the end he would beam when we clapped hands and applauded. It is not easy to teach Sam as he is still often reluctant to be shown sequences of notes on the piano or the xylophone although he clearly wants to be able to play tunes he knows. However, if he feels listened to, can sense that he is likely to quickly succeed, and there is still an element of fun and creativity, he is now more willing to briefly try. Laura has picked up Sam's special tunes and the way in which he can be helped to learn sequences, and has been able to use these ideas with him at home.

In general, Laura is warm and supportive in the sessions. She is clearly delighted with his enthusiasm, listening and taking part in sensitive ways. After the sessions, Laura and I discuss and reflect on what has happened while Sam plays with some toys. Sometimes we plan something specific for the following week, sometimes we just talk about the fun we have had and how Sam has drawn us into his creative music making. During the session the three of us have an easy non-verbal partnership and understanding.

In the next section I will reflect on the parents' perceptions of the sessions using themes that seem to have come out of Laura's and my descriptions of our work.

Original reasons for coming to music therapy

Laura thought that music therapy might be helpful to Sam because he had always enjoyed music. She mentioned that he was more engaged around music than in other situations and more cooperative when requests were sung to him rather than spoken.

Another parent, Gina, wrote that her son Luke had always responded to music and enjoyed making sounds. He would be calmed by music and would recognize tunes and copy part of them even before he could speak. He would tend to choose toys that made noises or played tunes. She also mentioned that Luke enjoyed listening to her husband playing the saxophone and the harmonica.

Heather wrote that it came as no surprise to her that her son Nick responded well to music as her husband was musical by profession. She told me that classical music seemed to help him to relax, and that he particularly loved it when his Dad picked him up and they moved together to the music.

Pat reported that the one thing she had always done for her son David was to sing. She would sing nursery rhymes and songs to settle him at night and to entertain him during the day. He seemed soothed by the rhythm and the predictability of the songs.

Karen was not sure that Peter would benefit from music therapy. However, she knew he liked music because he would dance and jump when he heard recorded music, and was delighted whenever she got her guitar out. She would also sing a little made up song to him every night at bedtime, which seemed to help him to relax and get ready for bed.

Although all these mothers are describing their sons' interests in music, they are also describing ways in which they and their families interact through music with the boys. The parents themselves are involved in the music making and it is perhaps partly because of their own enjoyment in the musical interactions with children with whom it is normally not so easy to connect, that they feel that music therapy is worth investigating.

Initial uncertainty

The referral procedure

Children at the Child Development Centre are usually referred to me by other members of the multidisciplinary team such as specialist doctors, clinical psychologists or speech therapists. Once I receive a referral I contact the family by telephone and suggest two initial assessment sessions. I explain that the sessions will last about half an hour, that the parent will be in the room with me and be invited to take part, and that we review the session together at the end while the child plays with some toys. I make it clear that at the end of the two assessment sessions we will decide together whether we think music therapy will be helpful and discuss what we feel our initial aims and objectives should be. Sometimes the families will ask me questions about music therapy over the telephone. I answer these but also indicate that they will have opportunities to ask further questions when I see them and that I will lend them a music therapy training video which should give them a good idea about the work.

The first sessions

Initially, the parents' first concern appears to be how their child reacts in the music therapy sessions and whether I will be willing to continue working with them. In addition, in spite of my explanations and the video, parents also express uncertainty about what their role should be.

Laura wrote that although Sam would run around in the waiting room, he would become very calm when I started to sing the 'Hello' song. In general she felt that the first session seemed to go well although Sam was not very cooperative. Later she wrote that at the beginning she had been unsure what her role would be in the sessions: 'I suppose I thought I was there to accompany Sam. I wasn't sure I would be joining in with the music making.'

Gina was also concerned at first, saying that initial sessions were quite difficult because she did not feel confident about what she was doing and Luke would get very angry. Heather reported that she had absolutely no idea what would happen or what Nick (or herself) would be expected to do: 'It was a bit of a surprise when after entering the room Amelia began by singing a welcome song. Were we expected to join in? Did we have to say anything? Was it OK for Nick to be making his own noises while Amelia was singing?'

Pat wrote: 'To be honest, I was disappointed after the first session–apart from a couple of moments where David seemed to let go and try something, he was mostly uncooperative and uninterested and there was no evidence of his love of songs and rhyme.' Karen was not sure what to expect at first: 'How could my son improve through music? How could music help him? At the first session I felt a bit awkward. Peter was given drumsticks which he received with a massive smile and I was given drumsticks which I received with perplexity . . . Was I expected to do something?'

Reading these accounts makes me wonder whether I am initially doing enough to explain about my work, and whether I should say more to parents about what their role will be within the sessions. How much I say when I first speak to parents on the telephone to arrange two initial assessment sessions varies from family to family and depends to some extent on how many questions I am asked and whether I have rung at a time when the person I am talking to has time to speak to me. My principal concern is to arrange a convenient time and place to work with the family but I almost always give a brief outline of what will happen. In addition, parents will borrow a music therapy training video between the first and the second assessment session.

Although I may explain that we will play instruments together and that parents will be invited to take part, perhaps it is not possible to convey what it *feels* like to communicate non-verbally through music making. However much verbal or written information I was to give to families it may be that until they are actually doing the playing themselves, the process of being involved in music making will come as a surprise. In some cases it may even be better for parents not to have time to think about this aspect of the work ahead of time, as it could make them feel more anxious or nervous.

One reason why it can be difficult to spell out exactly what will happen before the sessions start is that parents' roles in sessions will vary from one family to another, depending on the needs of the child, and whether younger siblings join in. The needs of the parents will also vary greatly, and the progress of the session may depend on what a parent feels able to contribute. In some cases all these needs and the parents' preferences will be very clear from the beginning of the work, in others only some aspects will be clear. In all cases needs and preferences will vary and change, sometimes from session to session and sometimes over longer periods of time.

Another theme that comes out of the comments about initial feelings about music therapy sessions is the concern that the child is not doing 'well' enough or showing me his real interest in music or how musical he is. I do tell all parents that the music making is a means to an end, but even so, parents come with the hope that the musical interests or strengths they have noticed in their child will be recognized.

Even though the children I see at the Child Development Centre are usually between 2 and 4 years old, most of the families I see will have already had many hospital appointments and seen a wide range of specialists to try to determine the nature of their child's difficulties. When they come to see me it may be the first time they are coming to see a professional about something they believe their child is good at rather than sharing an area of particular concern, so they are understandably disappointed if their child refuses to cooperate or does not do what they usually do at home. Again I think that all I can do here, after initial sessions, is to share my positive impressions, and state again that I am not expecting the child to behave well or perform in any way. Parents as well as children need time to realize that in music therapy sessions they will be accepted as they are, rather than judged or criticized.

Rejoicing in their child's enjoyment of the music

This feeling is common to nearly all the parents I have worked with and is written and spoken about at length by the parents themselves. It is also mentioned by many music therapists who have written about work with parents (Davies 2008; Drake 2008; Horvat and O'Neil, 2008; Loth 2008).

In a previous chapter that I wrote with Anna, one of the first parents I ever worked with, she wrote: 'It was a delight to be able to see John, who usually took no notice of anyone or anything for any length of time, become totally engrossed in making sounds and music. His enthusiasm and pleasure were so intense that it was impossible not to feel happy myself . . .' (Jones and Oldfield 1999 p. 168).

Gina wrote about Luke: 'Our music sessions have been a good way for Luke and I to try and manage his difficult behaviours because he responds so enthusiastically to singing and making music. We're both doing something we enjoy together.'

Pat expressed her own enjoyment even more clearly by writing: 'Most of all, I love to see him excited and enjoying himself and able to let go and join in.' Laura and Karen also write about their children's enjoyment but mention that they fell 'selfish' in some way. Laura wrote: '. . . being there, in the sessions, I can see that he loves to play the "rainbow bells" and the xylophones–he could never explain that to me. It may seem a little selfish, but I don't want to miss out on those special activities.' Karen wrote: 'I like to see Peter enjoy himself and learn through music . . . On a more selfish line, I like to feel that I am doing something to help him.' These feelings of guilt expressed by two such committed and devoted mothers surprised me. Children with autistic spectrum disorder are often puzzling and may not respond in usual ways to their parents. Karen had written that she had felt low and ineffective at times when looking after Peter, so music therapy sessions may have helped her to regain confidence in her own abilities. Perhaps both Laura and Karen sometimes became overwhelmed by attending to the special needs of their sons, and then needed a little support to allow themselves just to have fun.

It seems that it is the children's enjoyment that enables parents to feel happy themselves. The children's feelings are interwoven with the parents' feelings. When parents write about the music therapy experience and mostly describe what their child is doing or feeling, in some ways they are indirectly expressing what they themselves are experiencing. This brings to mind the famous quote by Winnicott (1964 p. 88): 'a baby cannot exist alone but is essentially part of a relationship'. Although the children I am working with are no longer babies, they are likely to be needier than children without specific difficulties. Often parents will have become more intensely involved with their child with special needs, in some ways making the bond between the parent and the child more like that of a parent and a baby.

The parents delight in their children's enjoyment of music and are also immensely proud of their children's musical achievements. One parent who had three older children as well as one 3-year-old boy with autistic spectrum disorder was quite tearful when he vocally completed sounds in a variation of 'Twinkle, Twinkle' in a very musical way. She said: 'I've felt proud of the other children before but never before of Ian in quite this way. His musical singing made me feel quite proud of him.' Pride was also mentioned by Laura who wrote that: 'Sam recently treated the family to a recital of 'Three Blind Mice' on the piano at home. There was much cheering and clapping and his little face just beamed with pride.' Many parents like Laura hope that their children may be able to access more 'formal' music teaching as they grow older. There are many extremely accomplished professional musicians with Asperger syndrome, so there is no reason why further musical education should not be possible for children on the autistic spectrum. Nevertheless, it is hard to predict which children will thrive musically even when they appear to be very musical at a young age. Although I am often very enthusiastic and excited about the musical abilities of 3 year olds I sometimes have to be careful not to raise expectations or create false hope for parents who may see musicality as one of the main strengths of their young child with autistic spectrum disorder.

Non-verbal interactions

Quite often in my work at the child development centre, I recreate opportunities for parents and young children with special needs to experience early non-verbal interactions. Most of the children will not have gone through the 'usual' babbling stage as babies, which means that the parents will not have had the chance to interact with their children through sound exchanges. Daniel Stern writes in detail about how parents can tune into their babies' moods through these babbling dialogues (Stern 1985, 1995, 1996). In music therapy sessions it is possible to recreate these types of exchanges through interactive music making, thereby providing not only an opportunity for the child to develop vocalizations and language but also a new way of communicating for the parent and the child.

Nevertheless, musical matching may initially seem very strange for parents. Although some parents find it easy to respond musically, others will need time to develop confidence. Often it is not so much the actual playing or singing that is hard but taking enough time to listen to what the child is doing and then sometimes waiting just the right amount of time before responding. The adult musical responses need to provide the right balance between imitating the child's musical contributions and slightly changing the responses so the dialogue remains creative and interesting rather than becoming boring. I will model these musical dialogues throughout the sessions in my music making with the children and the parents. In my verbal reviews with the parents after the sessions I might suggest specific ideas of musical interactions that can be explored at home, or I might suggest that sometimes a parent might want to pick up a child's musical idea rather than trying to get the child to copy the parent's idea.

Musical matching is something that needs to be experienced rather than explained, and in some cases parents need time to feel confident and at ease before these interactions can develop. In one case it took 10 months before a father I had been working with was able to take his son's musical lead. As the most important thing is for parents to feel relaxed and at ease it would be counterproductive for me to try and analyse and criticize parents who were 'mismatching' musically. In some cases of difficulty it can help parents to see excerpts of videos of the music therapy sessions. However, it is important to emphasize the positive aspects of the interactions between the parent and the child in these video reviews, particularly if parents lack confidence or are feeling low (Oldfield and Bunce 2001; Oldfield 2006b).

Many parents pick up new ideas from music therapy sessions. In questionnaires given to parents attending a music therapy group Loth reported that: 'Some parents rated seeing their child do new activities that could be used at home and finding different ways to interact with their child as the most important' (Loth 2008 p. 61). For parents who may have lost confidence in their ability to play with their children, being encouraged and supported to play musical instruments with their child could help them to regain some of that confidence.

Heather found that she gained confidence in music therapy sessions to then sing to Nick at home. She also reported that: '... Nick seemed to respond so well to music that his speech therapist was trying to convince his teaching assistant to sing him instructions when he needs to undertake a particular task.'

Peter enjoyed the sleeping game where he played instruments to wake me and Karen up. His enjoyment translated into starting to 'wake up' all the different members of his family at home. Although this was not always convenient, it was a positive sign of communication from a non-verbal and often quite isolated little boy.

Containing and addressing difficult behaviours

Many parents reported that they were anxious when their children did not conform or behaved in difficult ways. At the beginning Gina wrote that: 'Initial sessions were quite difficult because I didn't feel confident about what I was doing and Luke could get very angry.' Later she wrote: 'Over the weeks I've become less upset when he gets very angry. Being with him in sessions has helped in that we have both learned ways of dealing with his outbursts that I now use at home and when we are out and with groups of other people.'

Pat wrote: 'For me, music therapy is different because there is no pressure. David is totally accepted for what he is and we don't need to worry why he is like he is.' Both Laura and Gina found that their sons responded well to the: '1, 2, 3 ... finish' method of ending each of our activities within the music therapy sessions, and then successfully used this same method of finishing activities at home.

Karen and Pat mentioned that the predictable structure of the music therapy sessions seemed to be useful for Peter and David. This meant that they were able to create more predictable situations in other settings outside the music therapy room. Nevertheless, Karen needed reassurance after difficult sessions. She wrote: 'I like the fact that the music therapist always finds something positive to say about the session even if the whole session was spent trying to get him to participate.'

My role as a music therapist with the parent of a child who is not conforming, or is behaving in difficult ways, is first of all to make sure they are both safe, for example by quickly removing instruments that might be used to throw or hit. I then show that I am prepared to contain and deal with this behaviour and am not judging or accusing the child or the parent in any way. I try to discuss the difficulties with parents after the sessions. We attempt to understand why a child is misbehaving and then we decide together how to approach the problem. In many cases it might be best not to confront the child, but to compromise in some way. For example, recently a boy who we knew enjoyed being in the room with us made a point of refusing to come into the room at the beginning of the session. His mother and I made a game of this and sung a song while we carried him into the room in the chair he was clinging onto in the waiting area. This kind of technique can only be used within the context of a supportive relationship, and must be used thoughtfully, not applied to every similar situation.

On other occasions when a child may be making a point of refusing an instrument I am offering him, I will put that instrument aside saying: 'OK let's do something else now but later I would like you to play it.' Sometimes it might be a good tactic for the mother to play with me and for us both to ignore what might be an attention-seeking rebellion. However, there will of course be occasions when it is important to console a child who is genuinely upset or distressed and to provide a quiet nurturing atmosphere for that child. If a child is angry it may be possible to give them a chance to express this anger either by giving them and their mother loud instruments to play and/or by playing in very loud and angry ways myself.

Parents need lots of reassurance that I can accept difficult behaviours and indeed that I see it as our joint task to address and contain these difficulties. Once parents realize that I am not blaming or judging them in any way, we can work out strategies together, which parents can then use not only in the music therapy room but also at home and in other situations.

Working in partnership with parents

Initially I am often dependent on parents to physically guide their child or to help me understand their child's speech or special ways of communicating. Often parents will also need to be there to reassure their children. This supporting role is one that most parents feel at ease with and that helps the two adults to start working together. Sometimes a parent will be more or less direct with a child than I might be, but rather than criticize I feel it is usually better to accept the role they choose, and then gradually our joint working relationship evolves, and we may both be influenced by each other's way of approaching the child.

Heather wrote that: 'On a practical note I needed to be present simply to pick Nick up whenever he would choose to slump to the ground, or to stop him kicking his feet while sitting at the piano–thereby enabling Nick to concentrate more fully on the music.'

Karen indicated that, 'Initially the parent can act as a bridge between the child and the therapist, the relationship and trust between the child and the parent enabling some sort of connection between the child and the therapist . . .' Later she wrote: 'The success of music therapy somehow depends on the partnership between the therapist and the parent . . . They need each other to provide the best set-up for that particular child: the conjunction of the knowledge of the subject (music therapy) and the knowledge of the child. It needs to be a partnership.'

Horvat and O'Neil (2008) described a grandmother who took on the role of the co-therapist with the little girl with whom they were working. 'Lisa and Anna brought into the room the existing strength and closeness of their relationship. This itself introduced a new dimension to the work, their intimately attuned relationship being available to us all as a therapeutic tool.'

Conclusion

In this chapter, the parents themselves have shared their perceptions of what it is like to be in music therapy sessions and how they feel about the work. These thoughts have allowed me to explore the role that the music therapist plays with parents. Some aspects of this role are clear and the parents and I openly discuss ways in which we might expand vocal dialogues, for example, or how to approach a difficult behaviour. Other aspects are more subtle, such as gradually enabling a parent to trust me, or gently modelling alternative ways of communication through musical exchanges. Sometimes these exchanges will be talked about but at other times they will evolve through the experience of working together. Perhaps my role with parents is a little like the musical improvisations that draw us together. We have to be sensitive to each other's contributions while at the same time allowing the musical exchanges to flow, be unexpected and creative.

References

Davies, E. (2008). It's a family affair: music therapy for children and families at a psychiatric unit. In A. Oldfield, and C. Flower (eds) *Music Therapy with Children and their Families*, pp. 121–140. (London: Jessica Kingsley)

Drake, T. (2008). Back to basics: community-based music therapy for vulnerable young children and their parents. In A. Oldfield, and C. Flower (eds) *Music Therapy with Children and their Families*, pp. 37–51. (London: Jessica Kingsley)

Horvat, J. and O'Neill, N. (2008). Who is the therapy for?: Involving a parents or carer in their child's music therapy. In A. Oldfield, and C. Flower (eds) *Music Therapy with Children and their Families*, pp. 89–101. (London: Jessica Kingsley)

Jones, A and Oldfield, A. (1999). Sharing music therapy sessions with John. In J. Hibben (ed.) *Inside Music Therapy: Client Experiences*, pp. 165–171. (Gilsum, NH: Barcelona Publishers)

Loth, H. (2008). Music therapy groups for families with a learning-disabled toddler: bridging some gaps. In A. Oldfield, and C. Flower (eds) *Music Therapy with Children and their Families*, pp. 53–69. (London: Jessica Kingsley)

Oldfield, A. (2004). Music Therapy with Children on the Autistic Spectrum; Approaches Derived from Clinical Practice and Research. PhD thesis, Anglia Ruskin University.

Oldfield, A. (2006a) *Interactive Music Therapy–A Positive Approach: Music Therapy at a Child Development Centre*. (London: Jessica Kingsley)

Oldfield, A. (2006b) *Interactive Music Therapy in Child and Family Psychiatry: Clinical Practice, Research and Teaching*. (London: Jessica Kingsley)

Oldfield, A. (2008). Working in partnership and supporting parents. In A. Oldfield, and C. Flower (eds) *Music Therapy with Children and their Families*, pp. 19–36. (London: Jessica Kingsley)

Oldfield, A., and Bunce, L. (2001). 'Mummy can play too . . .': short-term music therapy with mothers and young children. *British Journal of Music Therapy*, 15, 27–36.

Oldfield, A., and Flower, C. (eds) (2008). *Music Therapy with Children and their Families*. (London: Jessica Kingsley)

Stern, D. (1985). *The Interpersonal World of the Infant*. (New York: Basic)

Stern, D. (1995). *The Motherhood Constellation–A Unified View of Parent-Infant Psychotherapy*. (New York: Basic)

Stern, D. (1996). The temporal structure of interactions between parents and infants: the earliest music? Unpublished paper presented at the 8th Congress of Music Therapy 'Sound and Psyche', Hamburg, Germany.

Winnicott, D. (1964). *The Child, the Family and the Outside World*. (Harmondsworth: Penguin Books)

Chapter 5

Evaluating parent–child group music therapy programmes: Challenges and successes for *Sing & Grow*

Kate E. Williams, Jan M. Nicholson, Vicky Abad, Louise Docherty, and Donna Berthelsen

Sing & Grow is an early intervention music therapy programme for families with children from birth to 3 years of age, who are socially, economically, or physically disadvantaged. It aims to improve parenting skills and confidence, promote positive parent–child interactions, stimulate child development, and provide social networking opportunities. Music and song activities are used in a therapeutic context to enhance parenting skills, improve parent–child interactions, provide essential developmental stimulation for children, promote social support for parenting, and strengthen links between parents and community services.

Introduction

The *Sing & Grow* programme was established in 2001 with a requirement of regular reporting against key performance indicators. Since the early years of the programme a number of evaluation approaches have been trialled and our successes have been critical for obtaining significant funding for the expansion of the programme nationally in Australia. Using *Sing & Grow* as a case example, this chapter discusses some of the common challenges in evaluation, and lessons we have learned from undertaking evaluation regularly. The authors of this chapter include three music therapists in *Sing & Grow* project management roles, and two academic researchers.

As music therapy provision for families with young children is a relative newcomer to the field of early parenting interventions, in order to be considered a viable alternative to other well-established approaches, it is essential that the effects of this approach are documented. In a climate where resources are limited, service providers are turning to research and evaluation when making decisions about funding programmes.

There is a clear imperative to undertake evaluation in projects such as *Sing & Grow*. However, music therapists may lack the time, research expertise or confidence necessary to undertake rigorous evaluations of their programmes. In order to address the need for evaluation of the programme, *Sing & Grow* sought a partnership with academic experts to create and implement an evaluation procedure.

Programme evaluation

Programme evaluation is a process of demonstrating whether a programme works or not. This includes gaining an understanding of who the programme works for, under what service-delivery conditions, and for which outcomes (Hauser-Cram et al. 2000). There are three broad types of evaluation: process, impact and outcome (Hawe et al. 1990; Green and Kreuter 2005). Each serves a different purpose and provides important evidence about programme effectiveness (see Table 5.1). Ideally, a process evaluation should be conducted first. This aims to determine whether the programme is being delivered as intended, to the client group of concern, and that it is able to be delivered to a consistently high standard, across clinicians, settings and over time. Once these things have been established, attention can turn to examining the impact and outcomes of the programme. Impact evaluation concerns immediate changes associated with the programme, while outcome evaluation examines longer term outcomes.

Evaluation can be a daunting prospect for clinicians. Conducting a high quality evaluation requires considerable effort. Barriers include time constraints due to workloads, pressures to provide maximum time in service delivery, and limited resources including money and personnel. Evaluations can also be threatening. Clinicians may fear the consequences should the evaluation indicate that the programme is not achieving its desired outcomes (Hawe et al. 1990). However, there are many important reasons for undertaking evaluations (Hawe et al. 1990). Evaluations can demonstrate that a programme is making a positive difference, and not inadvertently making things worse for clients. Evaluations can provide reassuring information about how

Table 5.1 Evaluation methods

Evaluation type	Key questions addressed
Process evaluation[1] Measures the activity and quality of the programme	Who receives the programme? (Reach)
	Who fails to enrol or fails to complete the programme?
	How satisfied are participants with the programme?
	How much of the programme is delivered? (Dose)
	How much of the programme is received by different participants? (Exposure)
	How well is the programme delivered, over time and across clinicians and settings? (Quality)
	How consistently is the programme delivered, over time and across clinicians and settings? (Integrity)
Impact evaluation[1] Concerned with the immediate effects of the programme (both intended and unintended). Corresponds with measuring the programme's objectives	Detail varies across programmes and designing the appropriate questions requires a sound understanding of the theory underpinning the programme. Broadly:
	Are programme participants showing positive improvements over the course of the programme on targeted behaviours or indicators?
	Are programme participants showing any adverse changes on target or other behaviours?
Outcome evaluation[1] Concerned with determining whether the programme has achieved its overall goal and longer term effects. Corresponds with measuring the programme's goals	Detail varies in the same way as for Impact evaluation. Broadly:
	Are any improvements in participants' behaviours maintained over the longer term?
	Are programme participants showing positive improvements in the long-term outcomes of interest?

[1] From Hawe et al., 1990.

well the programme is operating and enable identification of gaps that need to be addressed. Obtaining quality data about the benefits of a programme strengthens efforts to seek funding, recognition and other supports. Importantly, both positive and negative evaluation results improve an understanding of what works, contributing to both the development of the theory underpinning clinical practice and to the development of the profession itself.

Evaluation of parent–child music therapy programmes

How well does the practice of music therapy with the families of young children fare in terms of evaluation evidence?

This form of music therapy, particularly in a group setting, does not have a long and extensive history. While there is a developing literature describing parent–child music therapy programmes (Abad and Edwards 2004), evaluation research is notably limited. Published evaluations report that these approaches are associated with positive parent satisfaction (Oldfield and Bunce 2001; Abad and Williams 2007), improved parent–child interactions (Nicholson et al. 2008), enhanced child social and communication skills (Lyons 2000; Nicholson et al. 2008), and improved social support (MacKenzie and Hamlett 2005).

Overall, these studies provide encouraging evidence of the likely effectiveness of music therapy intervention with the families of young children. However, the majority of published studies were based on relatively small samples, repeated measurement of outcomes was rare, and few studies used measures with proven reliability and validity (Abad and Edwards 2004; Nicholson et al. 2008). It is clear that this field of practice still requires a period of development to allow for a robust research base to be established.

Introduction to the evaluation case study of *Sing & Grow*

Sing & Grow is an early intervention music therapy programme for families with infants from birth to 3 years of age, who are socially, economically or physically disadvantaged. It aims to improve parenting skills and confidence, promote positive parent–child interactions, stimulate child development and provide social networking opportunities. The programme involves 10, weekly group sessions for parents and children, conducted by music therapists. Music and song activities are used in a therapeutic context to enhance parenting skills, improve parent–child interactions, provide essential developmental stimulation for children, promote social support for parenting, and strengthen links between parents and community services (Abad 2002; Abad and Williams 2007; Nicholson et al. 2008).

An initial evaluation conducted by the clinicians involved data collection from 683 families attending 63 programmes in 2002–2005. Administrative data on programme delivery showed that performance targets were being met and the programme was provided to a wide range of disadvantaged clients, including young parents, single mothers, parents of children with a disability, and economically disadvantaged families. Parent-report measures indicated high levels of satisfaction (100% enjoyment; 94% would like to participate again), a positive perception of the programme's impact on parent–child relationships (70% reported feeling closer to their child); and a translation of activities to the home setting (87% used music for behaviour management

purposes at home). Therapist observations indicated that children were demonstrating improvements in their cognitive, physical and social development
over the course of the programme (Williams 2006; Abad and Williams 2007).

This initial evaluation had several strengths. The parent questionnaires were
reported to be non-intrusive and user friendly. Questions using a 'yes/no'
response format were easy to analyse and produced statistics that were simple
to communicate. Open-ended questions provided a richness of information
that was clinically useful, and clinicians' written records were used to illustrate
programme successes. Key limitations included an inability to demonstrate
changes over time (pre data were not collected on key outcomes), and the 'yes/
no' questions lacked the sensitivity that can be gained from scaled responses.
It was also planned that clinicians would observe and rate parent–child interactions during the programme. However the approach that was designed was
too complex and proved impractical. Despite these limitations, the results
of this evaluation were fundamental for securing further funding for the
programme.

Outsourcing versus using in-house 'know-how'

If researchers have the expertise in selecting research methods, data collection
and data analysis, why not simply outsource the evaluation? While this may
appear to be a simple solution that removes burdens from clinicians, this
approach is not recommended. Clinicians have expertise about the programme
and its clients that is essential for designing an appropriate evaluation (Hauser-
Cram et al. 2000). The best outcomes are achieved by a clinical–research partnership to maximize both sets of expertise at all stages of design, implementation
and reporting. Typically, it is recommended that researchers be engaged as
early as possible, and preferably during the programme planning stages
(Bamberger et al. 2004). However, time, effort, and resources can be saved if
clinicians undertake some background research first. This will assist clinicians
to gain a clearer picture of what they want from their evaluation, and can help
to clarify the research approaches that may or may not work with particular
client groups. Experience in collecting research data may also enhance the
clinicians' credibility with potential research partners (Hawe et al. 1990).

Step 1: Check whether you are ready for evaluation

Before engaging independent researchers it is important to check that the programme is ready for evaluation. A programme is 'ready' when it is possible to
demonstrate that it is reaching its target audience, it is being implemented
properly, clients are satisfied with the programme, and there is some evidence
of positive effects (Hawe et al. 1990). In this case, information was gathered on

each of these by the *Sing & Grow* clinicians, providing a good basis for proceeding to a more comprehensive evaluation.

Step 2: Allocate funding

The scope of an evaluation will be determined by available resources. Clinicians and researchers are seldom in the position where they can donate their time, so budgetary allocations are necessary. However, it can be difficult to secure funding just for the programme itself and service providers are often looking for ways to cut expenses. This presents a dilemma–evaluations can be costly, but in the absence of evidence that a programme is having desired effects, it may be vulnerable to cost-cutting. *Sing & Grow* endeavours to allocate 10% of the total programme funding for evaluation. It is not always easy to convince funding bodies of the importance of this. Publications and publicity that high-light the funders' role can help to ameliorate some concerns.

Step 3: Document your 'model of change'

In order to design an evaluation, it is critical to understand the theory that underpins the programme (Hauser-Cram et al. 2000; Bamberger et al. 2004). Programme theory (sometimes called 'programme logic') refers to the 'explicit theory or model of how the program causes the intended outcomes' (Rogers et al. 2000 p. 5). What is it that the programme is doing, that is leading to changes for participants? Sometimes there are clear documents outlining this, but often it is something that is implicitly understood, and needs to be elicited through consultation between programme developers and clinical staff (Bamberger et al. 2004). Developing an explicit statement of the programme theory is necessary for identifying what needs to be measured by the evaluation and to enable this to be articulated confidently to potential research partners.

Case study

Once the *Sing & Grow* programme was well-established, an action inquiry study was under-taken to examine alternative evaluation methods (Williams 2006). The main aim was to strengthen data quality through the use of parent-report measures with established reliability and validity. Potential measures were identified from the literature, and after discussion with leading academics, two questionnaire measures were selected. These were trialled with two groups of parents attending *Sing & Grow*. Structured feedback was collected from parents, clinicians, and staff from agencies associated with the programme.

The results clearly demonstrated that the selected tools were not optimal for evaluation purposes (Williams 2006). Key concerns included: that they were too long; the literacy level was too high for very disadvantaged clients; items were overly negative in their focus; some items were inappropriate for parents of very young children; and the measures failed to capture the full range of outcomes of interest. The timing of data collection was also a con-cern. Consistent with recommended practice for evaluation, parents were asked to complete the questionnaires at the start of their first *Sing & Grow* session. However, this reduced the time available for the programme, presented management challenges, for example having to keep children occupied while parents were filling in questionnaires, and was perceived to erode critical early opportunities for establishing clinician–client rapport.

Several lessons were learned from this early research. First, expert advice needs to be tailored to specific clinical contexts. This may not happen when the 'experts' are not closely involved with the programme, and tailoring requires an investment of time by the researchers. Secondly, off-the-shelf evaluation tools may save initial preparation time, but prove costly if the resulting data are of limited utility. The research also illustrated how an inappropriately designed evaluation can undermine therapeutic processes and alienate some clients.

This study clarified *Sing & Grow* requirements for the future evaluation and potential research partners. For example, the researchers needed to have or be prepared to develop a sound understanding of the specific therapy context; be sensitive to the characteristics of the client groups; and have the skills for identifying and/or modifying appropriate measurement tools.

Selecting, engaging with and maintaining research partners

Finding appropriate research partners can be challenging. There may be a limited pool of potential researchers with the relevant expertise and the capacity to take on new projects. There is no one obvious place to find researchers. Individuals with evaluation expertise may have backgrounds in the behavioural, social, health, or education disciplines and may work in university or other sectors. Before approaching potential research partners it is important to be well-prepared. We recommend the following six steps for identifying, engaging and maintaining relationships with research partners.

Step 1: Identify potential candidates

Use existing networks to find out who is doing relevant work in the area, talk to people who have worked with them before and examine publicly available documents about their work. The following questions are useful for guiding this process:

- Who is researching in parent–child early intervention?
- What is their professional reputation like?
- Are they flexible in their approach?
- What sort of research methods do they use?
- Do they have a reputation for listening and working well with people?

It may not be possible to answer all of these questions in advance, and some will only become clear once initial contacts have been made. However, from this scoping work, it should be possible to develop a shortlist of potential researchers to consider further.

Step 2: Prepare in advance of the first contact

When first contacting potential research partners, it is critically important to be able to clearly articulate:

- The nature of the programme to be evaluated–this may require provision of some background information about music therapy more broadly, as well as the specific nature of this programme.
- What sort of partnership is being sought–whether it is purely advisory or requires direct involvement; one-off or ongoing.
- The type of evaluation that is required–process, impact and/or outcome.
- The relevant timelines.
- The amount of funding available for the research.

As potential research partners will already have other commitments, it is crucial to convey not only professionalism, but also enthusiasm that is likely to capture their interest. It is essential that the researchers are aware from the outset, which aspects of the proposed research are fixed, such as non-negotiable reporting dates, and which are flexible. While the choice of a research partner will be guided by the researcher's relevant skills, ensuring complementary personalities is also important (Hawe et al. 1990).

Step 3: Discuss the potential costs and benefits to both parties

Clinicians and researchers work in quite different environments, that shape what work they do and how they approach this work. A successful partnership is one that maximizes the benefits for both partners and minimizes their costs. As a minimum, the following issues should be discussed (Hawe et al. 1990):

- What will the researchers get out of their involvement?
- How often will you meet?
- What sort of responsibilities will you share?
- What sort of responsibilities will you split?

Step 4: Clarify expectations and negotiate roles

Once a potential research partner has been selected, expectations and roles should be clarified. This requires attention to the relevant expertise of each party, as well as to potential competing demands. For academic researchers there are particular times of the year where their capacity may be quite restricted, for example when grant funding applications are due, or at the start and end of teaching periods. Some flexibility and negotiation may be required on both sides. Expectations and roles to be negotiated can include:

- Role descriptions and timelines–includes clarifying who will be responsible for collecting the data, cleaning and organizing it, entering it, analysing it, and reporting the findings.

- Data ownership and storage–who owns the data, where will it be stored and who will have access to it.

- Ethical issues–who is responsible for ethical clearance.

- Co-authorship agreements–who authors articles, how will an individual's role be acknowledged, and what defines contribution amongst an authorship group.

Step 5: Formalize the agreement

The chances of future misunderstandings and angst may be reduced by clearly documenting what has been agreed. Depending on the circumstances, a formal contract may be required. As a minimum, decisions made during meetings should be documented afterwards and circulated to ensure that there is shared agreement. While formal documentation will not prevent problems, for example if one party fails to deliver according to terms, it will facilitate resolutions.

Step 6: Open and frequent communication

Cross-disciplinary partnerships have inherent challenges. Partners bring with them explicit and implicit beliefs and expectations. Relationship development and maintenance requires careful nurturance. There needs to be adequate rewards for both parties if the relationship is to continue and prosper. Fundamental to this is clear, open and frequent communication. Face-to-face meetings can be challenging to organize, so phone and email contact is critical. Both partners need to keep each other informed of their progress, discuss challenges as they arise, and seek permission in advance for any public communications that acknowledge the other party (Hawe et al. 1990).

Case study

In 2004 *Sing & Grow* was funded for national expansion, which involved moving from a locally based programme to nationwide delivery. An independent evaluation was required as part of the funding contract. Potential research partners were initially identified by discussion with academic and community colleagues. After examination of research profiles and publications, three potential candidates were selected. An initial meeting was held with each separately, to discuss their potential interest and suitability according to the following criteria:

- Had an open and inquiring mind in regards to music therapy (none had prior experience with music therapy).
- Was willing to listen to and value the views of the *Sing & Grow* management and clinical teams.
- Recognized the vulnerability of the programme's clients and the need to place the least amount of burden as possible on them.
- Was willing to find creative yet valid ways of measuring programme outcomes.

One of the potential candidates (JN), when briefed about the nature of the programme, suggested including another colleague with complementary skills (DB). This demonstrated to the *Sing & Grow* team that a collaborative team approach, rather than a hierarchical one, could be possible. The initial interview included brainstorming some possible evaluation designs and discussion of what the researchers would want to achieve should they be involved with the research. Options for increasing resources through funding applications and student involvement were discussed.

A formal contract regarding roles, intellectual property, payments, and deliverables was drawn up by the lawyers from *Sing & Grow*'s host agency, and approved by the university legal advisors. The researchers drafted an initial document on authorship for papers and presentations, which was amended by the clinicians and agreed to. Proposed evaluation methods and timelines were negotiated in a series of subsequent meetings and formally documented in the researchers' first report to the funding body.

The relationship between the clinical and research teams developed in strength from the outset due to a number of factors. In a practical sense, frequent consultation during the early design and trialling stages, ensured 'ownership' by both groups. Less tangible, but of no lesser importance, was a sense of mutual respect for each other's expertise, a fortuitous match of personalities and work ethics, and a shared passion and curiosity for the work.

The benefits of establishing joint ownership and responsibility were considerable, and perhaps somewhat unusual. The researchers adopted the study as part of their core research programme. This enabled them to donate many unpaid hours to the evaluation, and they successfully sourced additional funding to supplement the evaluation budget by 50%. Attention to early outputs in the form of conference presentations and papers ensured that benefits were quickly apparent and allowed the researchers to justify their involvement to their respective employers.

Getting the right evaluation design and tools

The evaluation methods to be employed will be largely determined by the key questions the evaluation seeks to answer and the resources (funding and personnel) available. One benefit of a clinical–research partnership is that each party brings their own expertise and ideas about what is needed to advance the field. A collaborative approach can produce better design results than either would have achieved alone. However, to achieve a feasible and scientifically sound evaluation, a number of competing demands need to be resolved.

A first issue concerns data collection breadth and depth. Complex evaluations that seek to answer a number of questions (such as the one described in this chapter), require measurement of a wide range of constructs. Typically, it is not feasible to assess everything to the level of detail that would be desirable, and compromises need to be made. Our approach to this has been twofold: seek brief measures wherever possible; and ensure that key outcome measures are assessed optimally, but accept some compromises on other measures in order to reduce the amount of data collection. Comparability also needs to be considered. We selected key outcome measures that have been widely used, so that the resulting data can be compared with other studies. However, we also retained some clinician-designed measures to enable comparison with the results from earlier *Sing & Grow* research.

A related issue is client burden. The families who are most in need of early intervention are typically difficult to engage in services (Barlow et al. 2005). As illustrated earlier, collecting data from such clients can be burdensome and may potentially undermine their engagement with the programme. The evaluation design must therefore be matched to the capacity of clients by careful attention to the amount of time required to complete questionnaires, ensuring appropriate literacy levels and balancing positively and negatively framed questions.

The evaluation also needs to be designed so that it is appropriate to the service context, with methods that do not interfere with the quality of programme delivery. For example, where funding is provided for service delivery, it may not be possible to employ a control group design that would involve some clients not receiving the intervention. Alternative designs, such as matched waiting list control groups will need to be considered.

Some key steps we used to assist optimal evaluation design included:

- The researchers observing the programme to familiarize themselves with its normal procedures, staff skills and client characteristics.
- A continuous development and feedback process between the researchers and clinicians in relation to the overall design and specific measurement tools.
- Initial training and ongoing monitoring of staff responsible for data collection.
- A pilot period to trial methods and measures, with formal feedback processes to ensure that any problems were identified and resolved.

The evaluation of the national expansion of the *Sing & Grow* programme commenced with a 6-month pilot study in 2005 (Nicholson et al. 2008). The main evaluation was conducted during 2006 and 2007. A comprehensive evaluation was designed to assess process, impact, and outcomes, as summarized in Table 5.2. Table 5.2 also highlights some of the key findings to date (for more detail see Nicholson et al. 2008, 2010).

Table 5.2 Evaluation of the *Sing & Grow* national expansion 2005–2007

Key research questions	Measurement tools and source	Timing of data collection	Some key findings[1]
Process evaluation			
Were the target numbers of programmes and clients achieved?	Administrative data Managers' and clinicians' records	Once per programme	Targets met: 2379 families attended 242 programmes to September 2007
How much 'service' was provided? (Intensity)	Administrative data Clinicians' records	Once per programme	Ten sessions was not uniformly achieved: 21% of programmes had eight or fewer sessions
Who were services provided to? (Reach)	Parent report	Pre	Successfully provided to highly disadvantaged clients: 10% indigenous; 20% non-English speaking; 26% sole parent; 37% on government benefits
Who completed or failed to complete the programme?	Administrative data Clinicians' records	Every session	23% dropped out after 1–2 sessions
How well were services provided? (Quality)	Clinicians' ratings	Every session	Overall targets met, but with variations in quality by group size, client characteristics and geographical location
Impact evaluation			
Were there improvements from pre to post, in:			
Parents' mental health?	Parent report	Pre, post, 3-month follow-up	Significant decreases in mental health symptoms from pre to post; maintained to follow-up
Social support within each programme group?	Parent report	Post	98% reported the programme facilitated contact with other parents; 58% had contact with others outside the group

Parents' linkages with relevant services?	Parent report	Post	22% had contact with a specialist during sessions
Were parents using Sing & Grow at home?	Parent report	Post	87% used the Sing & Grow CD at home; 93% used music to have fun with their child
Were parents satisfied with the programme?	Parent report	Post	99% satisfied/very satisfied with the programme; 96% would attend again
Outcome evaluation			
Were there improvements from pre to post, and were these maintained over 3 months, for:			
Parents' parenting skills?	Parent report	Pre, post, 3-month follow-up	Significant increases in parental warmth and parenting efficacy, maintained to follow-up. Decreases in parental irritability, but not maintained
	Clinician observation	Sessions 1, 2, 9, and 10	
Children's developmental skills?	Parent report	Pre, post, 3-month follow-up	Significant improvements in child's social and communication skills, with further improvement to follow-up
	Clinician observation	Sessions 1, 2, 9, and 10	

[1] From Nicholson et al., 2008.

Engaging clinicians in research

Successful evaluations require the involvement of the clinical staff who deliver the programme (Hauser-Cram et al. 2000). Their roles may include: maintaining administrative records; encouraging client participation in data collection; collation of client data; and completion of their own observational or survey data. To engage in this process, clinicians need to be fully informed about all aspects of the research, its aims and potential contribution to evidence-based practice. Ideally there should be opportunities for staff to provide feedback and suggest improvements. Staff who feel their views are valued are more likely to be committed to the research, feel ownership of the process and make greater efforts to ensure high quality data collection.

There are considerable benefits in having clinical staff committed to the evaluation. Well-informed staff are better able to deal with client concerns about the evaluation, and to build rapport and trust with clients around the research process (Liamputtong 2007). If the clinicians are not committed, they will be less able to engage clients, and the data collection will reflect this. Clinicians who understand the research will be more confident in explaining how the clients' data will be used and its importance for future programme development and funding. This assists the clients, in turn, to feel comfortable in completing the evaluation tools, and not feel threatened when disclosing sensitive information.

Engaging clinicians in research also has potential benefits to professional development. Clinicians can gain valuable skills and knowledge of research processes and the administration and interpretation of evaluation tools. The importance of providing staff with adequate training and support for their role in the evaluation cannot be highlighted strongly enough. Training should include information about the:

- History and aims of the project.
- Rationale for the methods and measures being used.
- Importance of their role (and consistency) in data collection.
- Procedures for administering the tools.
- How the data will be analysed, and by whom.

To ensure that clinicians have the appropriate skills for their role, opportunities to practice and receive feedback on key tasks is advisable. Timelines for reporting the findings from the evaluation should be clear, with mechanisms in place to provide clinicians with regular progress updates.

Case study

When the *Sing & Grow* programme expanded to nationwide delivery (2005–2008), new management structures were established. This involved the appointment of eight full- or part-time staff with management and clinical duties, to oversee the workloads of 33 sessional clinicians. All received initial training on the *Sing & Grow* programme. This included information about the evaluation methods and their roles in data collection. Specific tasks were practised, such as how to explain the evaluation to clients. Videotaped examples of sessions were used to train clinicians to a consistent standard in rating client behaviours.

Ongoing supports included:

- A detailed evaluation procedures manual.
- A data management checklist of what was collected for each session.
- Ten per cent of sessions were attended by a senior staff member, who made independent ratings of client behaviours and the quality of clinician practice. These ratings provided a measure of reliability for the evaluation, and were also reviewed jointly by clinician and manager for clinical supervision purposes.
- Regular telephone contact and face-to-face meetings between clinicians and managers, and managers and researchers.
- At least annual group training days for all clinical staff.

In 2005, the evaluation methods were formally pilot tested. Management and sessional staff provided feedback on feasibility, appropriateness and where refinements were required. This gave all staff the opportunity to contribute to the shape of the final evaluation plan.

During the initial stages, concerns were expressed about potential workload burden. This was examined through interviews with the managers after the pilot study and questionnaires for managers and sessional staff at the end of the main evaluation. Qualitative comments from the managers indicated more positive than negative effects:

> It is good having someone . . . whose job it is to take care of [the evaluation]. It reduces my workload quite significantly. The [clinicians] also have less work . . . but they have to think a lot more about what they are doing and they have to be trained in it. It is getting people to think differently.
>
> [The evaluation] is very organised. You come out of a session and you take your book out and you just fill it out. It is very systematic. You do it each week. The [sessional staff] have not had any problems.

Questionnaire data from twenty sessional staff and all eight managers are summarized in Figure 5.1. These show that the most challenging aspect of the evaluation was the data collection in Session 1, rated as 'difficult' by 43% of staff and 'very difficult' by a further 11%.

> The evaluation at the start is challenging because there is so much to take in [during] that first session. Just remembering names and whose child belongs to whom was challenging [enough] . . . let alone [rating] the quality of the interaction for each dyad.

However, all other aspects of the evaluation were rated as 'easy' or 'very easy' by 70–85% of staff. While three of the managers reported that it was 'difficult'

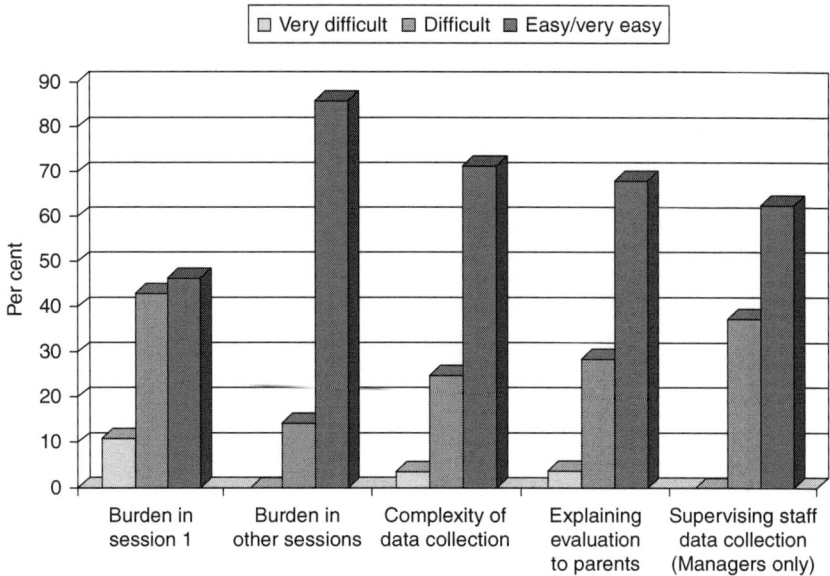

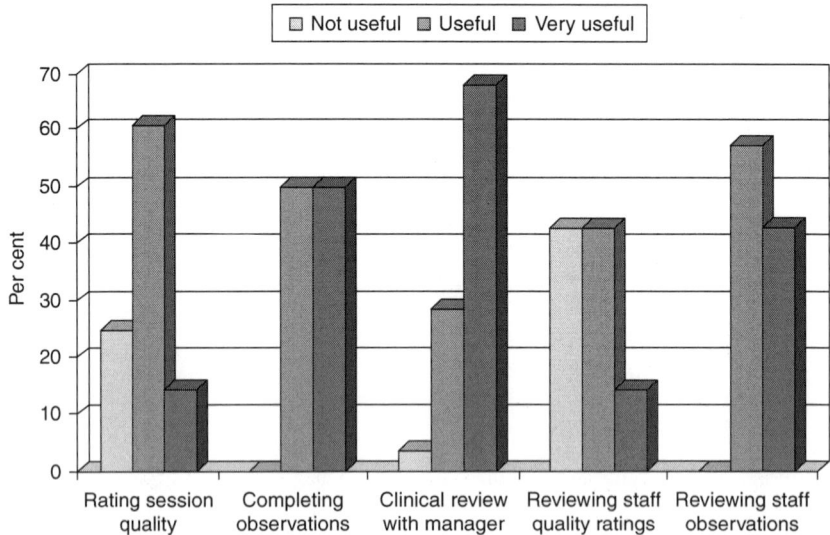

Fig. 5.1 Staff and managers' ratings of the burden and usefulness of the evaluation methods.

to oversee the data collection of their staff, the remainder described this as 'easy' or 'very easy'. The evaluation tasks designed to facilitate clinical supervision, received mixed reviews: 25% reported that the ratings of session quality were 'not useful', whereas there was almost unanimous agreement that the parent–child observations were 'useful' or 'very useful' for clinical practice.

Overall, these findings suggested that the evaluation did not impose an unreasonable burden on staff. Moreover, the collaboration between the evaluation team and *Sing & Grow* resulted in the development of evaluation methods that were also useful tools for the supervision of clinical practice. As one staff member commented in her questionnaire:

> Even though the evaluation was a hassle at times, it did become easier . . . and I recognise it as a fantastic opportunity for music therapy and it also helped me reflect on the responses [to the programme] of the families involved.

These findings also shaped subsequent changes. In 2008 when the programme was granted a further 12 months funding, client questionnaires (particularly for Session 1) were shortened, administrative data collections were simplified, and the frequency of collecting quality ratings was reduced.

Conclusions

Since the first evaluations of early childhood interventions were published in the 1960s, 'there have been lively debates about the usefulness and limitations of quantitative evaluations' (Hauser-Cram et al. 2000 p. 487). It is hoped that the example provided here has illustrated many of the potential benefits that arise from a well-designed evaluation that combined the strengths of both qualitative and quantitative methodologies. Designing the *Sing & Grow* evaluation was an interactive process between the researchers and clinicians. The researchers brought to this process an extensive knowledge of published measures and related research from non-music therapy disciplines. The clinicians contributed points of advocacy from staff and client perspectives regarding the accessibility and usability of the tools, and were able to prioritize which outcomes were the most important to measure. As a result, the final design and data collection tools were developed by consensus. It would not have been possible for either team alone to have designed such a comprehensive, appropriately targeted, yet succinct, approach. Both groups acquired new knowledge and skills from this collaboration.

Based on our experiences with *Sing & Grow*, and informed by other writers in the field of evaluation (Hawe et al. 1990; Bamberger et al. 2004), we have identified the following as critical factors for the development of a successful clinical–research partnership:

Shared power. Careful selection of the research partners is needed to ensure a good match in terms of philosophies and theoretical approaches, and to enable the development of a partnership (not a consultation) process.

Shared control. Clinicians and researchers bring different and necessary expertise to the evaluation process. It is essential that both parties' views and concerns are taken into account, especially in the early stages when procedures and methods are being developed.

Shared goals. Ongoing consultation is essential to ensure a good match between the research and clinical goals. Negotiation of outputs such as publications and presentations (including who will take lead authorship, what type of journal or conference to submit to, and timelines) is useful for ensuring that there are benefits evident for everyone.

Shared accountability. Related to this, it is also critical that the researchers and clinicians are aware of and meet the obligations of their relative roles. The clinicians need to have a clear understanding regarding the importance of collecting high quality data, while the researchers need to be attentive to non-negotiable things, such as timelines for deliverables. Both will potentially be required to commit to extra efforts to ensure the smooth running of the project.

Legitimate independence. Researchers need to be aware of the clinicians' professional responsibilities to their service and clients. In turn, the clinicians need to be aware of the researchers' responsibility to objectively interpret their findings, and the ethical use of research data (e.g. not divulging identifying information).

Mutual respect. It is important that differences in expertise, philosophies and needs are recognized and valued. This includes being considerate of each other's competing demands and being willing to take on additional responsibilities from time to time.

Open and regular communication. Problems invariably arise in long-term projects. Open and regular communication enables the early identification and resolution of challenges. Provision of regular feedback allows all relevant parties to discuss emergent findings and provides opportunities for ongoing programme development. This can facilitate continued engagement and enthusiasm at all levels. By avoiding 'nasty surprises', good communication is also fundamental to ensuring shared control and mutual respect–for example, keeping each other informed about planned absences, and seeking consent or feedback regarding the content of publications and presentations.

Evaluations that provide quality data about the effectiveness of clinical practice not only enhance the profile of the music therapy profession, but also improve the likelihood of attracting future funding. Our experience with a clinician–research partnership allowed our programme to remain accountable to the funding body by monitoring the implementation of the project against its stated aims. From the perspective of the clinicians, the collaboration was a valuable journey. Exposure to the evaluation enhanced the practice of the clinicians' involved and increased awareness of the impact that the programme could have. It provided an exciting opportunity to see their work contributing alongside more traditional and established disciplines such as family therapy, psychology, and social work.

Acknowledgements

National expansion of *Sing & Grow* was funded by the Australian Government Department of Families, Housing, Community Services and Indigenous Affairs (FaHCSIA) under the *Invest to Grow* and *REACh* initiatives. Findings and views reported are those of the authors and should not be attributed to FaHCSIA. JN was supported by a National Health and Medical Research Council Career Development Award (ID 390136). The authors thank the Playgroup Associations in Australia, especially Playgroup Queensland, the agencies who supported the programme, and participating parents and children.

References

Abad, V. (2002). *Sing & Grow*: Helping young children and their families grow together through music therapy early intervention programs in community settings. *Annals of the New Zealand Society for Music Therapy*, 2002, 36–50.

Abad, V., and Edwards, J. (2004). Strengthening families: a role for music therapy in contributing to family centred care. *Australian Journal of Music Therapy*, 15, 3–17.

Abad, V., and Williams, K. (2007). Early intervention music therapy: reporting on a 3-year project to address needs with at-risk families *Music Therapy Perspectives*, 25, 52–58.

Bamberger, M., Rugh, J., Church, M., and Fort, L. (2004). Shoestring evaluation: designing impact evaluations under budget, time and data constraints. *American Journal of Evaluation*, 25, 5–37.

Barlow, B., Kirkpatrick, S., Stewart-Brown, S., and Davis, H.T.O. (2005). Hard-to-reach or out-of-reach? Reasons why women refuse to take part in early interventions *Children and Society*, 19, 199–210.

Green, L.W., and Kreuter, M.W. (2005). *Health Program Planning: an Educational Andecological Approach*, 4th Edn. (New York: McGraw-Hill)

Hauser-Cram, P., Warfield, M.E., Upshur, C.C., and Weisner, T.S. (2000). An expanded view of program evaluation in early childhood intervention. In J.P. Shonkoff and S.J. Meisels (eds) *Handbook of Early Childhood Intervention*, 2nd Edn, pp. 487–509. (Cambridge, UK: Cambridge University Press)

Hawe, P., Degeling, D., and Hall, J. (1990). *Evaluating Health Promotion: a Health Worker's Guide*. (Sydney: MacLennan and Petty)

Liamputtong, P. (2007). *Researching the Vulnerable: a Guide to Sensitive Research Methods*. (London: Sage)

Lyons, S.N. (2000). 'Make, make, make some music': social group work with mothers and babies together. *Social Work with Groups*, 23, 37–54.

MacKenzie, J., and Hamlett, K. (2005). The Music Together program: addressing the needs of 'well' families with young children. *Australian Journal of Music Therapy*, 16, 43–59.

Nicholson, J.M., Berthelsen, D., Abad, V., Williams, K., and Bradley, J. (2008). Impact of music therapy to promote positive parenting and child development. *Journal of Health Psychology*, 13, 226–238.

Nicholson, J.M., Berthelsen, D., Williams, K., and Abad, V. (2010). National study of an early parenting intervention: Implementation differences on parent and child outcomes. *Prevention Science*, 11, 360–370.

Oldfield, A., and Bunce, L. (2001). 'Mummy can play too. . .': short-term music therapy with mothers and young children. *British Journal of Music Therapy*, 15, 27–36.

Rogers, P., Petrosino, A., Huebner, T., and Hacsi, T. (2000). Program theory evaluation: practice, promise and problems. In P. Rogers, T. Hacsi, A. Petrosino, and T. Huebner (eds) *Program Theory in Evaluation: Challenges and Opportunities*, pp. 5–13. (San Francisco: Jossey-Bass)

Williams, K. (2006). Action inquiry into the use of standardized evaluation tools for music therapy: a real life journey within a parent-child community program. *Voices: a World Forum for Music Therapy*. Retrieved 17 November 2006, from http://www.voices.no/mainissues/mi40006000208.html.

Chapter 6

The benefits of music sessions for very young children with their parent or carers through the eyes of a music therapist

Margareta Burrell

A little girl is sitting in anticipation, eagerly waiting for the session to start, observing the room and the instruments. From the CD player in the corner, she can hear African music. In comes a mother with a toddler and a baby, discussing where they are going to sit. The toddler immediately spots the drum and runs to it. He plays it with gusto and then turns it upside down to see what is inside. The other little girl observes him with great interest, but is too shy to join him in his explorations.

Making music in open and informal groups at Coram Parent Centre, UK, allows the possibility to include families from a multitude of cultural and social backgrounds. These groups can focus on the healthy and normal child and parent, while the leader makes use of the opportunity for early observation and assessment of any special needs. In close collaboration with Centre staff and specialist services, it is possible to point parents and their children to additional supports when vulnerability is observed.

Music and movement to support parent–infant interactions

Music and movement sessions have been provided as part of a drop-in pro-gramme at the Coram Parent Centre in Camden, London since 2000. Over the last 50 years Coram has developed the concept of the Children's Centre, now well established all over Britain, as a place where education and health needs for young children and their parents and carers are met under the same roof. The Centre provides a Nursery School for 3–5 year olds, a Day Centre for infants from birth to 3 years, a Parent Centre Drop-In, as well as a range of services provided by specialists and therapists. Coram is also specialized in the provision of adoption services.[1]

The Parent Centre welcomes all families with children 3 years of age or younger. The Centre is a place for learning and connecting with others and also a place to receive support, not only for the children, but also for the adults. Many opportunities arise for parents to get involved in further training, social activities, and job opportunities. Above all they are encouraged to enter the world of young children, bringing with them a range of cultural and social backgrounds with various expectations about their child's development, education and health.

As an early years music specialist, a qualified music therapist, and a Dalcroze teacher, my approach is informed by the combination of my training and work experience, as well as having had three children of my own. These different elements have been integrated to inform my music making in this community setting, where I also teach children and staff in the day centre and nursery and organize musical events and workshops. I work part-time as a music therapist with individual children and their parents at different times of the week. The fact that I am not British gives me further credibility in this multicultural environment as I have had to learn all the traditional rhymes and songs and adapt to the British way of life myself.

My training as a music therapist means that my focus is on the child's emotional development and well being. The field of music therapy has increasingly become aware of the functions of attunement and attachment as a basis of a healthy relationship for the very young child between his/her mother, parent and carers (Stern et al. 1985; Trevarthen 2002; Gerhardt 2004). Music is an easily accessible and highly sophisticated means for communication, interaction and expression. Through engaging in musical improvisations a sense of togetherness and closeness emerges and can be observed and supported. As relationship is at the centre of human well being music making with the very young and their parents seeks to enhance, balance and strengthen all of their skills of relating.

Music therapy offers partnership through sensitive musical play. Musical play is direct in its emotional impact and yet it is flexible and creative. Musical play provides a basis for the parent and infant to explore their way of being together and to develop skills of relating to each other (Trehub et al. 1997; Stern 2000). Finding ways to practice and perform rituals of relationship in the early years is essential to the development of skills of relating that can 'determine

---

[1] www.coram.org.uk.

relationships of affectionate attachment, trust and companionship, and defend against abuse, mistrust and disregard, [which] are fundamental to the ecology of emerging human consciousness' (Trevarthen 2002 p. 171).

During these early years, patterns of behaviour and relationship are apparent when working with babies and toddlers. The way we model respectful communication and playful interactions with them can have a positive and preventative influence in developing the emotional capacities of both the child and the parent (Papoušek and Papoušek 1981). Through musical play, led by the child and supported by the parents, the emerging relationship deepens and the patterns of behaviour are enriched and expanded. This process happens not only through the involvement in the sessions, but also through the mutual observation of each other of the many and varied couples present.

A typical session

The children's buggies are parked in front of the Centre in rows and the children are playing in the garden of the Children's Centre. The adults are standing and chatting and overseeing the many adventures with tricycles, sandpit, water play or painting. Others are playing with the children. In the room, some are playing with lentils and pots and pans, others are exploring a basket full of treasures with cones and brushes and spoons to shake, tap and feel. The twins are sitting in the corner with their Nanny, who is reading them a story. The play worker is chatting to a mum about her sleepless nights. The music leader is calling for her session to begin shortly.

In the room next door the small chairs are set up in a big circle. Music is greeting the children. A little girl is sitting in anticipation, eagerly waiting for the session to start, observing the room and the instruments. From the CD player in the corner, she can hear African music. In comes a mother with a toddler and a baby, discussing where they are going to sit. The toddler immediately spots the drum and runs to it. He plays it with gusto and then turns it upside down to see what is inside. The other little girl observes him with great interest, but is too shy to join him in his explorations. The twins are arriving. They want to sit as closely to their nanny as possible and all settle down. Now many other children with their parents start to arrive and quickly form a circle. At the door is a dad with his toddler. His son is reluctant to come in and would rather carry on playing on the tricycle. Dad stays at the door with him, comforting him and distracting him by talking about the guitar and the accordion in the corner.

The session is starting and all eyes and ears focus on the hello and welcome song. The ritual is familiar and all join in. Now everyone is full of anticipation about what is to come.

The door opens and a little boy comes running in, followed by his father. The boy heads straight for the guitar the leader is playing. In no time the boy is strumming the strings with his hands. He moves towards the bag of instruments to explore its contents. He seems oblivious that a great number of eyes are on him in amazement. His father manages to find a place to sit and invites the boy to join him. The leader invites the group to stand up and offers a basket with many coloured ribbons on sticks. Soon everybody in the room dances to the music from the accordion, making the ribbons swing and fly and turn. Our little boy has listened, too and manages to sway his ribbon together with the other children to the music. The father seems pleased and joins his son in some helicopter swirling. As the music changes, the ribbons soon adapt to the calmer music and start to sway and gently rock. After a lively dance, including some jumping, turning and stamping, the group is exhilarated; some children are quite excited.

A tune is heard form a bamboo pipe and all activities stop. All eyes are fixed on the source of this sound. The children are drawn to it; some reach out for the pipe. The mood changes and all calm down, listening and focusing. Some children go back to their parent and sit on their lap, being gently rocked. Others are swaying with their bodies. Not a word has been spoken, but the music has provided the cues for a change of response.

Typical responses

Joshua sits on his mother's lap; he is about 2 years old, so this is appropriate. He listens carefully, observes everything around him, and takes part with the help of his mum. He never makes a sound. He does not speak; he does not dare to leave his mum; he is very shy.

His mum brings me photographs of Joshua at home. He is sitting on his little chair, holding a toy vacuum cleaner playing it as if it is a guitar. Joshua is attempting to sing every song we have learnt.

The Balafon with the two chunky beaters makes glorious sounds. It is easy to play and takes any amount of banging and tapping. The beaters are being passed from one soloist to the next, while the 'orchestra' is playing shakers. Ruby has been chosen to be the leader, pointing to whom she decides to play. She can also make everybody 'stop' and wait, before they are allowed to 'go!'

Syd is 2 years old and loves to play the drum. He moves towards the drum whenever he has an opportunity. After many moments of exploration, touching and turning the drum, examining the inside and the sides, he finally discovers how to play it. He does so with both hands, alternating, then together, playing loudly, quietly, on the skin, but also on the sides. He has a strong and regular beat and is totally absorbed while playing. His mother watches him with amazement. She says she has never seen him taking initiative like this in order to express himself. He can normally only stay engaged with any activity for a brief moment. Here he is giving a real performance.

Zara, a little girl of 3, is looking through the window at the door while the music session is going on. She is pulled by the sounds she can make out, observing eagerly where the music is coming from and what goes on in the room. She is waiting for an opportunity to slip in and be part of it, when an adult finally opens the door. Her mother is with the baby and reluctant to come in. In her culture, music and movement are not something done in public, especially for a woman. Zara comes in at the first opportunity and stands right in front of me. Although she does not really understand any English, she copies everything I say and do precisely, observing every movement, listening with her whole being, totally absorbed in what is going on. She is communicating and interacting with me and laughing when she understands. For several weeks afterwards, Zara seeks out the music sessions. Her mum eventually joins her, baby on her lap, sitting in the background observing, but later joining the group and starting to partake in the activities. Even when Zara leaves to go to nursery, she returns with her mother and the baby to all of the sessions.

In a letter from a mother (2003)

> I cannot begin to tell you how much we have enjoyed our music sessions over the last 18 months . . . in fact our lives have revolved around the Wednesday morning sessions.

Tom loves his music. He may be shy in class, but at home he sings, plays flute, piano and drums. Our songs make queues bearable and train rides calm. We will always cherish and remember when Tom first came to his love of music.

Supporting social development

These music groups are considered 'open' as anyone can take part. Parents bring their children in the hope of giving their child a head start in future education, high achievement and well being. They bring their child to have fun and to be entertained, or to establish a firm foundation for any musical talents. However, the added benefit is that music can become an inspirational part of daily life, giving parents permission to 'play' with their child.

The playful context of making music with young children is often light heart-ed and quite casual. This is not an overtly clinical or therapeutic context but the relevant ingredients for therapeutic processes are present and at work. Positive attachment is encouraged and supported, while a secure and safe environment of respect and affirmation is modelled. The parent is learning when to hold back and to observe, when to respond and affirm, and when to stimulate and to encourage. Firm and safe boundaries create a trusting environment, within which there is room for improvised and free expression. Both child and parent can enjoy getting to know and respect each other in this creative and satisfying process. Music can catch a child's attention and imagination, engage them, invite them to focus and concentrate, motivate them to communicate and learn, and encourage them to order their movements and regulate their emotions.

As the group is large, comprising up to 10 couples, it demands clear boundaries and direction. Changing and varying activities with a good pace, as well as some rituals and repetition of songs and activities help to maintain a clear structure, making it safe and familiar. Within this structure there is a lot of room for improv-isation and input from the children and parents. Any contributions are welcomed, responded to and affirmed; other times they help as a distraction from negative behaviour. Ideas are picked up and copied, often providing encouragement to develop confidence and leadership for all members. We sing traditional and new songs, in the appropriate voice range and accompanied on a variety of instru-ments. We sing in different languages. We do actions with our hands and body.

Group music making requires the use of social skills. For many infants these music sessions are often the first time they find themselves part of a group. For first or only children especially, their own desires and wishes are central to everyday life at home. In this group context there are many demands to make contact, to relate, to interact. Parents probably find this just as hard as their children. They have little control over how their child will respond and 'perform' and can feel quite vulnerable, as their young children are not easily persuaded or manipulated. Parents can support, encourage and model; some let the child make progress on their own, others don't have the patience to wait and respond for the child.

One of the most beneficial outcomes in the situation is the way the parents learn from each other. They are able to observe, as well as compare, copy and learn from others how to set boundaries and how to engage with their child. The group often carries and supports the adults just as much as the children. Exchanges between parents before and after the session can help to reduce anxieties and provide a network in which they feel included and supported.

The therapist provides music that facilitates models and encourages the interactions, but it is the parent who has to respond, interact and communicate with the child in those early days and develop a 'secure base' for relationship (Bowlby 1983). In a group this becomes a simple task as it is easy to join in and copy others. As we repeat all the songs and activities, all become more confident and assured. Music can become a part of the daily routine of communication for each member of the relationship. For example, in the baby group, babies lie on mats on the floor. The adults are shown how to tease them with a song that involves placing one finger gently all over their bodies, singing 'Spot, spot, spot, spot . . .' and then 'stripes', 'buttons', and so on. This song can be sung during nappy changes helping the infant to tolerate discomfort and providing an opportunity to use the time for intimate and engaging play.

Supporting musical development

There are many musical elements present in the simplest nursery rhyme. Learning these builds the child's repertoire of songs and becomes part of a child's music and language development. Through this musical exposure the child builds a strong sense of pulse and meter, phrasing, form, dynamics, accents, crusis and anacrusis, pause and then climax. Experiencing a range of tonalities, modes, melodic patterns, and harmonic changes, all contribute to a successful encounter with music.

Musical elements have to be presented to both children and the parents as simple and contrasting ideas such as fast and slow, stop and start, loud and quiet. These basic musical elements give a structure to many of the group's musical games. Simple percussion instruments are available and the children learn to take care of them and to play them in the appropriate way. Movement around the room in response to musical signals is also part of the routine. We negotiate the space, getting to know each other by dancing in different groups.

Supporting the resolution of difficulties

During the many varied and contrasting activities, patterns start to emerge. Gentle and non-judgemental observation gives insights into the needs of the child, the parent and the couple. Problems become easily apparent in this welcoming setting. Interaction between the parent and their child—even after many invitations—can be non-existent, leaving the child exposed, confused and vulnerable. Some children seem almost invisible, as the parents are taking control of each and every attempt of the child's responses. Sometimes the exhaustion on some parents' faces tells the story of sleepless nights and the tedium of daily routines.

Musical interactions can successfully support attunement behaviours (Trevarthen 2002). Musical games demand full attention and concentration. Adult and infant are present for each other, interested, respectful, and eager to get to know each other's wishes and needs. This musical relating deepens the bonds of love, which are essential to human well being at all stages of life.

Sam

Sam, aged 12 months, is anxious and does not want to come into the room. He screams when his father brings him in. They stay outside the room and look through the window in the door. After 2 weeks of watching from outside the room, Sam can tolerate standing with his father on the inside of the door. His dad lets him observe and no pressure is apparent. During each of the following sessions, Sam gets closer and closer to the circle where the others are sitting, until he sits there with all the others. His father has supported him successfully.

David

David is not used to sitting on his mother's lap. He knows that his baby brother has got that place firmly and almost permanently occupied. David finds it hard to concentrate and keeps wandering about. He asks for a drink in the middle of a song.

Later he takes the instrument the girl next to him has and plays with it. She wants it back, but David does not want to give it back. When his mum calls him, he ignores her. She takes the instrument from David and gives it back to the girl, which so angers David that he lashes out. He then throws himself on the floor and cries. Thankfully we can distract him and let him play the big drum with the huge beater. He beams again.

Lily and Arif

Lily sits on her mother's knees, facing her. They sing 'Row, row, row your boat', a game the mum used to play with her mother, and her grandmother had probably played with her also. Later they say a rhyme, which requires some answers from Lily: mum invites the answers by giving intense eye contact and by the way she uses her voice. Much nodding is occurring and the bouncing is building up to a climax when Lily anticipates that she will fall safely between her mum's knees, accompanied by laughter and the word 'again!' Arif would like to play that game, too. His mum hesitates in putting him on her knees—when they see how much fun Lily is having, Arif and his mother join in.

Luke

Luke is looking serious. He does not take part, nor does he manage to smile. He is unresponsive and looks uninvolved. When offered an instrument, he leaves it on the floor in front of him. Mum sits behind him, without taking part. She seems in a world of her own and is unconcerned about Luke's isolated state and lack of interest. Is she depressed? Is Luke depressed? It will be important to talk to her after the session to try to make contact and to gently enquire as to how they are getting on. A little girl goes over to Luke, picks up the instrument in front of him and hands it to him with an encouraging smile and spontaneous sense of loyal support, inviting him to join our playing.

In considering the interactions with Luke, it is often not the right moment to attempt anything more than making a gentle observation. However, a picture of a child's safety, health or well being can quickly emerge. If there are concerns, staff are alerted and discussions take place. There is a possibility to refer the child to a specialist such as the music therapist, or to the psychologist or to a support worker. Early diagnosis is always helpful in order to set up a networked support system. Attending the weekly music sessions can then often offer some continuity and normality while parents negotiate the world of therapy and medical assessment and care.

Goodbye

As the circle is formed and starts to move with the music, it symbolizes the inclusive and essential sense of community, which can be created through the music and the movement. Some children go to the centre of the circle and dance their own dance. Some parents lift their child and dance together. Many have broad smiles on their faces when the dance comes to an end.

A lullaby gives a chance to calm down and to experience some rocking and swaying while cuddling and holding. The Bamboo pipe perfectly supports these actions with its mellow and clear sound. We end with a goodbye song:

... bye, bye, bye! Thank you for the listening; thank you for the singing; thank you for the dancing! We'll see you next week!

References

Bowlby, J. (1983). *Attachment*, 2nd Edn. (New York: Basic Books)

Gerhardt, S. (2004). *Why Love Matters.* (Hove: Routledge)

Papoušek, M., and Papoušek, H. (1981). Musical elements in the infant's vocalization: their significance for communication, cognition and creativity. In L.P. Lipsitt (ed.) *Advances in Infancy Research*, Vol. 1, pp. 163–224. (Norwood, NJ: Ablex)

Stern, D. (2000). *The Interpersonal World of the Infant: a View from Psychoanalysis and Development Psychology.* (New York: Basic Books)

Stern, D., Hoffer, L., Haft, W., and Dore, J. (1985). Affect attunement: the sharing of feelings states between mother and infant by means of inter-modal fluency. In T. Field and N. Fox (eds) *Social Perception in Infants*, pp. 249–268. (Norwood, NJ: Ablex)

Trehub, S.E., Schellenberg, E.G., and Hill, D.S. (1997). The origins of music perception and cognition: a developmental perspective. In I. Deliége and J. Sloboda (eds) *Perception and Cognition of Music*, pp. 103–128. (Hove: Psychology Press)

Trevarthen, C. (2002). Making sense of infants making sense. *Intellectica*, 34, 161–188.

Chapter 7

Supporting attachments in vulnerable families through an early intervention school-based group music therapy programme

Karen Kelly

Lena tended to sit facing away from her mother during sessions, observing others in the group rather than participating. She shrugged her mother away when she encouraged her to participate in songs or musical games with her. Lena's mother continued to be very encouraging in sessions by modelling actions, smiling, and initiating eye contact. Gradually Lena's participation began to increase. She could choose instruments with encouragement from the therapist and her mother, began to follow directions, and joined in with action songs. In the final session of the programme Lena stood up with the other children and turned to face her mother. Lena and her mother smiled as they faced each other for music making together.

Introduction

The programme is a family-based music therapy programme offered in schools in Limerick city, Ireland. Families experiencing risk and vulnerability due to their social, geographic and economic circumstances have the opportunity to participate in a series of weekly music therapy sessions. This Irish school-based music therapy group programme was provided for the needs of marginalized or at-risk families.

The Blue Box Creative Learning Centre is a charity organization that provides creative arts therapies services to schools in Limerick city. Services include music therapy groups at preschool and primary school levels, and individual music therapy and art therapy sessions at primary and secondary school levels; the aim is to help children reach their full potential through the creative arts therapies (Blue Box 2007). The Mission and Vision of The Blue Box Creative Learning Centre is:

> To bring about real and lasting social and cultural change by developing emotional and psychological supports and making them available to young people and their families within their communities. To this end, to make Creative Therapies available and affordable where the greatest need exists. (Blue Box 2007)

Regeneration

Limerick city has an unemployment rate five times the national average, a high proportion of one-parent families, a high crime rate, and many of its citizens experience significant educational disadvantage (Fitzgerald 2007). A number of Limerick-based organizations have a stated mission of meeting the needs of vulnerable families. For example, the Limerick Regeneration Project (LRP) was set up as part of a National Development Project in Ireland that works towards 'building communities through regeneration' (Limerick Southside Regeneration Agency 2007).

One of the key objectives of the LRP is to create a more balanced social mix in social exclusion areas. It highlights the important role of schools in tackling social exclusion and improving access for communities. Some of these children display difficulties with speech and language, concentration, gross and fine motor skills, and sensory attachment. The LRP proposes that children living in regeneration areas should have the best quality preschool provision, which must include active learning, as well as cognitive, language and social development. The promotion of home-learning and parental involvement is also emphasized in their mission. Early childhood services have a key role to play in children's emotional and social well-being and preparing them for successful experiences in formal schooling. The LRP has proposed that parent and toddler groups should be provided with resources to offer support to parents and children, and that therapeutic services could be developed in settings that are comfortable for both parents and children.

> There needs to be greater support for parents to assist them with their responsibilities for their child's development and upbringing. It is important to recognize that parents are the greatest influence in their child's development. Any supports should focus on

nurturing a positive relationship between parent, child and the wider family. (Limerick Southside Regeneration Agency 2007)

It is in this context that the need for the programme and its eventual provision has been developed.

Needs of the families

Living in circumstances of social deprivation can have a significant impact on parental stress, with many parents enduring extreme financial problems, difficult home lives, and depression. These circumstances have a profound effect on both their own lives and the lives of their children.

The author has observed that some parents also experience low self-worth, especially in relation to their parenting skills. This may particularly be the case for single or teenage parents. The challenges faced by these parents can be experienced by the baby's grandparents also, who can often become a child's primary caregiver when teenage parents are either no longer able to cope or when they are required to take up work, including in some cases relevant to work available in the area, extensive shift work. A wide range of social supports are needed for vulnerable families, including immigrant families from the refugee and asylum seeker communities who are settling into Irish society under challenging circumstances.

The role of music therapy to support parent–infant bonding

A number of reports have proposed the value of music therapy to promote positive parent–child interaction in group settings (Oldfield 1995a, 1995b, 2006; Shoemark 1996; Trolldalen 2000; Oldfield and Bunce 2001; Abad 2002; Abad and Edwards 2004; Rykov 2004). Music programmes led by qualified music therapists address the needs of vulnerable and at-risk families, including those with low income, single parents, young parents, those with drug and alcohol addiction, those with disability, and members of cultural minorities (Abad and Edwards 2004). Rykov (2004) proposed that music programmes for at-risk mothers and infants have an important and unique role to play.

Edwards et al. (2007) described how infants of refugee and asylum seeker mothers in Ireland often experienced anxiety and stress from a young age, and how positive interactions and closeness were often infrequent or even absent in many of the interactions between these preoccupied mothers and their children. Weekly music therapy groups were offered to mothers in the asylum seeking community who were caring for their young children in hostel accommodation and/or rented community dwellings. Case descriptions showed how the music therapy group was a time for the mother to focus exclusively on her child, and for children to have an experience of affectionate, attentive play (Edwards et al. 2007).

There is a developing literature suggesting that where social exclusion and marginalization is present mothers can find it difficult to interact or bond with their child (Oldfield and Bunce 2001; Oldfield et al. 2003). Music therapy can therefore be used successfully in enhancing the parent–child relationship.

Music therapy has also been used in promoting interactions between depressed mothers and their infants. Seiner and Gelfand (1995) observed that when mothers pretended to be withdrawn with depressed affect, toddlers physically withdrew from them, made more negative physical bids for attention, and became more unfocussd. When the mothers displayed normal mood states the toddlers were more positive, played closer to their mothers, and were never unfocused. Field (1998) demonstrated that depressed mothers exhibited fewer positive faces, and fewer animated faces and voices. Infants of depressed mothers produced more sad and angry faces and showed fewer expressions of interest. They also showed less exploratory behaviour (Field 1998). This research is important as it shows that the caregiver's ability to provide an emotionally available and regulated environment for the infant affects the infant's behaviour positively.

Music therapy provides musical interactions that are accessible to both the parent and their infant, encouraging the exploration and maintenance of positive and successful interactions between them. Rykov (2004) noted that at-risk parents, especially teen parents, may need to learn how to sing to their child, what to sing, and why. Through carefully designed activities in a group programme, caregivers and their children are brought together in a subtle but effective way.

Programme description

The programme was originally implemented into specific preschools in the Limerick city area. These schools provide free preschool education to families living within so-called 'disadvantaged' areas, by targeting children from 3 to 4 years of age who are at risk for failing to reach their potential within the education system (Citizens Information 2008).

The programme is provided by the Blue Box Creative Learning Centre to schools within the socially vulnerable areas of Limerick city, providing families with equal opportunities to avail of services which encourage a healthy family relationship, without any financial cost for the families. The programme described here was run in selected schools for between 8 and 10 weeks, and aimed to strengthen family relationships and develop children's social, cognitive and physical skills. It also offered opportunities for increasing confidence, reinforcing school concepts, and increasing and developing the children's language skills.

Sessions were run by qualified music therapists, including the author, and usually took place in the preschool classroom. Weekly 45 min sessions offered opportunities for parents to share interactive play time together with their children, enhancing their relationship within a musical context. When a parent could not attend the sessions, it was arranged that another close relative would attend the sessions instead. It was emphasized to parents that the children must be familiar and comfortable with the person who accompanied them to the sessions due to the content of the sessions and the aims of the overall programme. Sessions needed to be held in a friendly, comfortable environment and they needed to be accessible and fun.

The music therapy groups led by the author usually consisted of an average of 10 dyads, depending on class sizes on the day. The programme was offered to all families in the preschool classes. A diverse combination of family members and cultural backgrounds was a prominent feature of the groups. For example, within the groups there were single mothers, stay at home dads, older siblings, aunts, grandparents, and families of three or four nationalities. The teachers usually remained within the groups for the sessions. They acted as models for families during sessions and were also on hand to offer assistance to caregivers and to the therapist when necessary.

Parents were encouraged to arrange babysitters for younger siblings for the duration of the sessions as the programme was intended for the school child only. It was envisaged that younger siblings would attend the preschool in the future and therefore would gain the benefits of the music therapy sessions at the time. Although, when parents did bring another sibling to sessions the teacher assisted that infant so that the parent was free to focus their attention on the school child. This allowed the school child to get the most benefit from the sessions.

Session format

A basic format was used in each session in order to foster anticipation and familiarity with the sessions structure from week to week. This predictability of the session format was intended to help the children become familiar with routines. Children began anticipating certain aspects of the sessions, such as specific types of interactions, and the returning of instruments to the therapist at the appropriate time.

At the same time it was also necessary to be flexible with the format of sessions, so each session could be adapted by the therapist to suit the needs of a particular group. For example, the inclusion of the children's own ideas and suggestions often altered the session structure. Sessions always began and ended in the same way, starting with the 'Hello' song and finishing with the 'Goodbye' song. The rest of the session could be adjusted as required.

Session description

The group sat in a circle for the sessions. Caregivers sat on chairs and the children sat on cushions on the floor in front of them. This meant that the children were at eye level with their caregivers when they stood to face them.

The activities used in the sessions were designed to promote positive interactions between these dyads. Face to face interaction was encouraged along with hand over hand assistance, sharing instruments, gentle physical touch, hugging and kissing, instrument playing and singing together. Sessions also included fine and gross motor actions, and relaxation and movement to music.

The therapist modelled actions for caregivers at first to stimulate group participation. This was often a more successful way to encourage participation rather than expecting caregivers to be creative in initiating ways of using music and interacting with their children. Oldfield (2006) described how she often found it more useful to demonstrate or model activities rather than give lengthy verbal explanations.

Each session began with the 'Hello' song, acknowledging all of the families' attendance at the group. The song allowed for the children to respond verbally to the therapist, offering opportunities to build confidence in group situations. It also provided humorous moments as caregivers watched and listened in anticipation for what their child would say when asked through song how they were today. The 'Hello' song was also a good 'icebreaker', with children in the group telling the therapist each other's names. Some children took a few weeks of observing the therapist before interacting with her or participating in the session. This response most likely reflected their meeting of new people in their own social environment.

After the 'Hello' song, the children were encouraged to stand and face their caregivers, which prompted face to face interactions early on in the sessions. The pairs participated in hand clapping songs, tickling each other and rubbing noses. These actions facilitate positive interactions and are designed to promote the development of healthy relationships.

Families that already had a strong relationship were good models of positive behaviour for other dyads during these activities. The therapist offered direction on ways to participate in the sessions through the words of the songs, but also included opportunities for families to be more expressive once motivated to participate.

The use of instruments in sessions offered the children opportunities to develop their social skills through activities that involved listening, waiting, turn-taking, leading and following directions. Children waited their turn to choose instruments, followed directions for when and how to play, and listened to other group members playing. Children also learned to share instruments with each other. Children who had initially held tightly to an instrument or cried when requested to share began to swap their instrument with other children in the group so that another child had a turn of that instrument. Some children also began to share instruments with their caregivers.

Opportunities for children to increase and develop their language skills were also incorporated into the sessions. Through greetings, singing, imitating sounds, and naming instruments children exercised their language skills.

Caregivers assisted children in reinforcing concepts learned in school such as colours, counting, body parts, animals, sounds, and shapes. They helped their children with holding up the correct number of fingers during fingerplay songs, identifying shapes and colours, and pointing to correct body parts during gross motor action songs. Children were also encouraged to count their caregivers' fingers. In the song 'Heads, Shoulders, Knees and Toes' caregivers provided hand over hand assistance when children pointed to their caregivers' body parts. Parents/caregivers are seen as being the most influential people in a child's life and the most important thing here was that caregivers were interacting with and assisting their children. This offered caregivers opportunities for increased self-esteem, especially those who had limited education.

The group sessions offered various opportunities for increases in confidence for both the children and their caregivers. Shy caregivers began to interact more with other families, while children demonstrated increased choosing of instruments and verbal interactions. Some caregivers who attended the programmes displayed signs of low self-esteem and were often observed to be 'hiding' behind their children in sessions. The sessions aimed to provide a non-judgemental, safe environment for these families where they could explore and develop their relationships. Children sometimes offered encouragement for their shy caregiver, smiling at them and demonstrating ways for them to use instruments.

Conducting activities provided children with the experience of leadership. Children were asked by the therapist to use their arms to instruct the other group members for when to play or when to stop. 'Conductors' were usually first assisted by their caregiver, who provided hand over hand assistance from behind, and later conducted the group on their own. Children gained a sense of control over the group while the other group members cooperated by following the leadership skills of the conductor. As conductors became more confident they began to speed up or slow down the tempo of the music, much to the amusement of the other group members. Group members' confidence also grew through playing solos and duets. Caregivers often looked proudly on as their children grew in confidence playing for the group, with smiling faces. Children who had originally stared blankly when offered instruments to play in the first session, were now standing up and playing confidently for others to see and hear. Caregivers also became more confident, joining the children in playing duets for the group.

Both caregivers and children followed gross motor actions in response to the words of the songs. Some caregivers participated in doing the actions or dancing with their children during gross motor activities, while others found it amusing to observe their children dancing, laughing and wiggling to the music. One parent commented that she just enjoyed seeing her child so happy. The song 'Dingle Dangle Scarecrow' encouraged children to cuddle into their caregivers while waiting in anticipation to jump up and shake around, at the amusement of the adults in the group. Some caregivers kept their children on their laps and used them like 'puppets' moving their children's arms and legs for them at the appropriate time, the children giggling on their laps.

Nearing the end of each session caregivers were encouraged to sing to their children in activities that also promoted slow movements to music such as rocking and swaying together. Well-known songs such as 'Row Your Boat', 'In Dublin's Fair City', and 'You are my Sunshine' were used to encourage participation from families. It took a number of weeks for some adults to begin to sing to their child. As the weeks progressed caregivers' singing increased, creating a comforting environment for families to connect and bond. Each session then ended with the 'Goodbye' song where families were thanked for attending, and encouraged to attend the next session.

Developing expertise in relating through music

The following clinical examples illustrate some of the benefits experienced by families during music therapy. Notably an increase in positive interactions was observed and more successful initiation and completion of joint activities.

Increased face to face interaction occurred between one mother and child

Lena tended to sit facing away from her mother during sessions, observing others in the group rather than participating. She shrugged her mother away when she encouraged her to participate in songs or musical games with her. On occasion she slapped her mother, followed by a smile when she gained her mother's attention. In their first two sessions Lena pushed her mother away when she offered Lena assistance or tried to do face to face actions with her. Even so, Lena's mother continued to be very encouraging in sessions by modelling actions, smiling, and initiating eye contact. In the third session they attended together, during an action song Lena's mother leaned over her daughter's shoulders to do the actions with her, at which Lena responded to by smiling and doing the actions. In the sessions that followed

Lena's participation slowly began to increase. She began to choose instruments with encouragement from the therapist and her mother, began to follow directions, and joined in with actions to songs. Her hostile responses towards her mother also decreased. In the final session of the programme Lena stood up with the other children and turned to face her mother. Lena and her mother smiled as they faced each other for music making together.

An increase in one mother's confidence in sessions resulted in increased interactions between her and her son

Both Johnny and his mother presented themselves in sessions as appearing shy, pale and tired, and often unkempt. They tended to arrive late to sessions and did not interact with other families before leaving. During initial sessions Johnny's mother tended to observe other mothers before participating with him. She appeared to be shy during sessions, lowering her head behind Johnny, who she kept on her lap facing away from her. She smiled on occasion when Johnny participated in activities or spoke to the therapist. From her third session her level of participation increased. She slowly began to model actions, offer verbal prompts, provide assistance, and sing quietly behind Johnny. As her confidence in sessions increased so too did her interactions with Johnny, which appeared to occur more naturally and spontaneously. She also began to smile much more in sessions, especially when Johnny turned around to look at her. Increased gaze between mother and child was observed, along with playful interactions while sharing instruments, such as tickling, and laughing together.

Feedback from the classroom teacher indicated that Johnny's mother was experiencing extremely difficult circumstances at home, which sometimes prevented Johnny from attending school and often left his mother socially isolated. The teacher described how Johnny's mother 'came out of herself' in the sessions, and had told the teacher how much the sessions meant to her and Johnny.

One girl's language increased and developed during the programme

Sarah, a child with language difficulties, tended to imitate the sounds she heard around her during sessions. She would mimic sounds other children made and say one-syllable words, such as 'bye' and 'hi', when waving to or greeting the therapist. Sarah would sing or hum along to the songs in sessions, and when requesting an instrument she would either sound out the first letter of the word or try to say the colour of the instrument. Any sounds made by Sarah were encouraged and praised by the therapist. As the sessions progressed, Sarah's use of language increased and became clearer through greetings, singing, imitating sounds, and counting. Through the repetition of naming instruments she began to verbally communicate to the therapist which instrument she wanted. Nearing the end of the programme she said 'lollipop drum', which was acknowledged by the other caregivers in the group. Sarah also began to say the names of other children in the group, singing 'hello' to them during the 'Hello' song and welcoming families when they arrived to the sessions.

Music stimulated positive interactions between a preschooler and his mother

Evan attended the sessions with his mother. Evan's mother presented herself in the sessions as being low in mood, appearing tired and unkempt, and displayed unanimated facial expressions. This flat affect was seen on her son's face also. During sessions both Evan and his mother tended to sit and stare at other families rather than participate or interact with each other. When the therapist spoke to Evan he gazed at her. Evan and his mother did participate in some face to face activities though tended to do the actions while looking past each other or looking at other families. With some gentle encouragement from the therapist and teacher Evan's participation began to increase, which increased even further when his mother's level of participation increased.

By the end of the programme Evan and his mother still seemed a little uncomfortable with face to face activities although they had come a long way. The sessions in this case stimulated more positive intimate interactions between Evan and his mother.

Increased affection between one girl and her grandmother

Jenny's grandmother accompanied Jenny to the sessions. When Jenny misbehaved or refused to participate in activities with her she made jokes to make light of the situation. She mostly observed Jenny during sessions, offering praise when necessary. As the programme progressed Jenny's grandmother's encouragement towards Jenny increased. She began to offer Jenny assistance and even started to model actions to songs. On the occasions when she did not offer assistance Jenny turned around to look for her grandmother, and smiled when she gained her attention. Jenny's behaviour towards her grandmother had begun to change. Both became more affectionate, participating fully in face to face activities and smiling at each other. In the final two sessions Jenny's grandmother was observed by the therapist to be singing to Jenny during quiet time. She hugged Jenny and even gave her a kiss, which Jenny responded to by giggling.

Support was offered by a father for another parent in the group

Daniel and his father William were from a non-Irish background. At the start of the programme William sat quietly during sessions offering support for Daniel by smiling towards him when he participated in activities. Father and son attended each week and soon William's level of participation increased. When Maria, a single mother, was experiencing difficulties with her son Michael in the sessions William began to assist her by offering direction to her son and encouraging him to be good for his mother. His gentle manner encouraged more appropriate behaviour from Michael, who was lacking a father figure in his life. From then on the two families sat next to each other in sessions, and Maria appeared more comfortable in sessions with William's support.

Evaluating the programme

Eighty dyads attended sessions over one academic year. The sessions were evaluated in a number of ways; through written evaluation, written and verbal feedback from teachers, and through surveys of caregiver participants. The evaluation procedure monitored various behaviours that occurred during sessions such as children's skills, levels of participation, levels of interaction, and eye contact between dyads. The evaluation findings are based on evaluations received from 60 of the caregivers who participated, and feedback from the classroom teachers.

Feedback

It was important to get feedback on the programme so that it could be adapted and developed to best suit the needs of the families. Each teacher was requested to provide written feedback following the running of the programme with their class. They were asked to comment on any changes in behaviours between family members and any specific improvements that they noticed in the children's skills. They were also encouraged to share suggestions for improvement to the programme.

Liaising with teachers before and after sessions proved invaluable in giving feedback, gaining information about families, and sharing observations made during sessions. Teachers often reported to have seen relationships develop and strengthen during the sessions. One teacher expressed how it was nice for her to see families sharing the sessions together and looking happy considering the difficult home lives they were experiencing.

Another teacher described how it was a great opportunity for her to see how the caregivers and children interacted within a different context. She also described how she observed changes in some caregivers' attitudes towards the school and towards their children's education in general. She told how some parents had difficult experiences in school themselves, many of which had been in the same school as their child, and as a result seemed to have a 'block' about entering the school. As parents became more comfortable being in the classroom with their children, they also seemed more comfortable entering the classroom at other times.

Teachers commented on the social interaction they observed between Irish and non-Irish families. They pointed out that non-Irish mothers were beginning to speak with other caregivers in and outside of sessions and had even started to create friendships. Teachers described how they saw shy caregivers appearing more confident with their children in sessions. Many of the teachers also reported to have seen improvements in the children's social skills, especially with waiting, turn-taking and sharing.

Feedback from caregivers was gained in two ways: through conversations with the therapist and/or teacher directly after sessions; and through written feedback requested by the therapist in the form of a short survey.

The mother of one little boy approached the music therapist after a session to thank her for 'improving his confidence and self-esteem'.

Surveys were given to caregivers at the end of each programme. The teacher distributed and collected the surveys after the music therapist had left and read through the questions with the caregivers so that any queries could be answered. Caregivers were given the option of completing the survey in the classroom or to take it home for completion. The following confidential survey responses were collected over a year and a half of running the music therapy programme and indicate that the programme was considered beneficial by those it was intended to support.

The survey responses revealed that 97% of caregivers reported that their children had enjoyed the sessions, and 97% of caregivers reported to have enjoyed sharing the sessions with their children. Eighty-five per cent of caregivers indicated that their relationship with their child strengthened during the programme. Eighty-eight per cent of caregivers noticed an improvement in their children's skills while attending the programme. Eighty-seven per cent of the families began to use music more at home following their attendance of the programme, and 97% of caregivers would recommend the programme to others.

Caregivers were asked to comment on which aspects of the programme they liked best. There were three main themes that emerged from their responses: (a) the music; (b) the social aspect; and (c) the interaction between caregivers and their children. Caregivers' comments indicated that they enjoyed the musical aspect of the sessions through 'singing', 'dancing', and playing a 'variety of instruments'. Responses regarding their relationship or interactions with their children suggested that caregivers showed awareness of how the programme may have benefited them. Comments that caregivers made when completing the surveys included; 'being with my child', 'spending 1:1 time with my child', 'to see how he developed in the last few weeks', 'watching my child's confidence grow', and 'to see the children smiling and so happy'. Caregivers also recognized the social benefits of attending the programme with comments such as having 'opportunities to meet other families'.

Conclusion

The programme provided opportunities to strengthen family relationships between preschool children and their caregivers living in socially vulnerable circumstances. The programme was reported by teachers and caregivers to have improved the quality of relationships between caregivers and children. Relationships were nurtured and the development of stronger bonds was observed. Shy caregivers began to offer direction and assistance to their children in sessions, while others began to allow their children the freedom to explore within a safe environment. Caregivers who had initially observed their children struggling during activities began to assist and support them. Additionally, parents and children already experiencing a healthy reciprocal relationship had opportunities to reinforce and further strengthen their bond. During the programmes caregivers learned new ways of interacting with their children, and both the children and their caregivers gained new skills that they could share together in the sessions and at home. The programme was also found to be effective in improving the children's social, physical and cognitive skills. Children learned to wait their turn, share with others and build confidence. They exercised their coordination skills and practised and increased concepts learned in school, with the support of their caregivers. The programme offered social support for families and opportunities for caregivers to play a more active role in their children's education.

Observations made by the therapists during the sessions suggested that a follow-on programme may be beneficial for the families. That programme was later developed and implemented into the same schools, offering families the opportunity for developing and reinforcing benefits achieved in the first programme.

References

Abad, V. (2002). Sing & Grow: helping young children and their families grow together through music therapy early intervention programmes in community settings. *Annual Journal of the New Zealand Society for Music Therapy*, 36–50.

Abad, V., and Edwards, J. (2004). Strengthening families: a role for music therapy in contributing to family centred care. *Australian Journal of Music Therapy*, 15, 3–16.

Blue Box (2007). The Blue Box Creative Learning Centre. Available at http://www.bluebox.ie/images/updocs/annual%20report%202006.doc. Accessed 19 August 2008.

Citizens Information (2008). Early childhood education. *Citizen's Information Board*. Available at http://www.citizensinformation.ie/categories/education/pre-school-education-and childcare/early_childhood_education. Accessed 21 June 2008.

Edwards, J., Scahill, M., and Phelan, H. (2007). Music therapy: promoting healthy mother-infant relations in the vulnerable refugee and asylum seeker community. In J. Edwards (ed.) *Music: Promoting Health and Creating Community*, pp.154–168. (Newcastle-upon-Tyne: Cambridge Scholars Publishing)

Field, T. (1998). Maternal depression effects on infants and early interventions. *Preventive Medicine*, 19, 200–203.

Fitzgerald, J. (2007). *Addressing issues of social disadvantaged areas of Limerick city: Report to the cabinet committee on social inclusion.* (Limerick: Limerick Regeneration Agency)

Limerick Southside Regeneration Agency (2007). *Our Community, our Vision, our Future. Regeneration of Southill and Ballinacurra Weston.* (Limerick: Limerick Regeneration Agency)

Oldfield, A. (1995a). Communicating through music - the balance between following and initiating. In T. Wigram, R. West, and B. Saperston (eds) *The Art and Science of Music Therapy: a Handbook*, pp. 226–237. (London: Routledge)

Olfield, A. (1995b). Music therapy with families. In T. Wigram, R. West, and B. Saperston (eds) *The Art and Science of Music Therapy: a Handbook*, pp. 46–54. (London: Routledge)

Oldfield, A. (2006). *Interactive Music Therapy in Child and Family Psychiatry: Clinical Practice, Research and Teaching.* (London: Jessica Kingsley)

Oldfield, A., and Bunce, L. (2001). 'Mummy can play too . . .': short-term music therapy with mothers and young children. *British Journal of Music Therapy*, 15, 27–36.

Oldfield, A., Adams, M., and Bunce, L. (2003). An investigation into short-term music therapy with mothers and young children. *British Journal of Music Therapy*, 17, 26–45.

Rykov, M. (2004). The lullaby group program: Descriptions and development. Available at http://www.musictherapy.ca/docs/confproc/2004/rykov.html. Accessed 12 March 2006.

Seiner, S., and Gelfand, D. (1995). Effects of mother's simulated withdrawal and depressed affect on mother-toddler interactions. *Child Development*, 15, 19–28.

Shoemark, H. (1996). Family-centred early intervention: music therapy in the playgroup programme. *Australian Journal of Music Therapy*, 7, 3–15.

Trolldalen, G. (2000). Music therapy and interplay: a music therapy project with mothers and children elucidated through the concept of 'appreciative recognition'. In J.Z. Robarts (ed.) *Music Therapy Research: Growing Perspectives in Theory and Practice*, Vol. 1, pp. 74–86. (East Barnet: British Society for Music Therapy)

Williams, K. (2006). Action inquiry into the use of standardized evaluation tools for music therapy: a real life journey within a parent-child community program. *Voices: a World Forum for Music Therapy*. Available at http://www.voices.no/mainissues/mi40006000208.html. Accessed 7 January 2007.

Chapter 8

Music therapy to promote attachment between mother and baby in marginalized communities

Joanna Cunningham

The mothers supported their babies on the edges of their laps. I tilted my head down to the babies and sang, looking into their faces. I accompanied my singing on a classical guitar using a finger picking style in 4/4 time. It was a warm and soothing musical environment and each baby, regardless of age or severity of condition, looked into my eyes and held my gaze unwaveringly until the pause after the final chord. Following the 'Hello' song I sang the babies' names over and over improvising with tempo, rhythm and melody. Each of these interactions lasted around 5–7 min during which the remaining group members watched and listened as the music reached into the baby, the mother and the space between them and for that moment held them.

Introduction

This chapter provides a description of my experiences as a mother, a music therapist, and a musician. It moves through and between the professional and the personal and, using these worlds, attempts to explore and describe how music can move through the space between a mother and baby and ignite a miraculous bond.

This account is comprised of a number of explorations followed by an examination as to how the discoveries outlined can be brought to the most vulnerable in our community. The first of these explorations, simply, is the acknowledgement that music is a part of us either consciously or unconsciously. Music exists as a reflection of what it is to be human. As a species we cannot but make music; it is the form we have found to harness the abstract musical elements that exist in everything from the rumblings at the earth's core to cycles or rhythms which support every time frame. The second relates to the unique relationship between mother and baby followed by a description of my witnessing and facilitating as a music therapist while offering my music and sounds to the mother and baby. These sounds are put into the world of this pair in the context of the music therapy session and used to unlock the euphoria which, when released, flows and gushes and floods into the dynamic space between the two beings.

Music therapy for parents and their infants with Down's syndrome: the music in us all

In the earlier part of my career as a music therapist I worked with a group of mothers and babies. The babies were diagnosed with Down's syndrome and all were under 12 months of age. Seven pairs attended a weekly group music therapy session. The session was around 45 minutes in length. The mothers sat on chairs in a semicircle with the babies on their knees and I sat on a chair in front of them with my guitar. We began the session by singing hello. I pulled my chair close to each mother and baby in turn and sang to them:

> Hello, hello, hello to you,
> It's good to see you today, today.
> Hello, hello, hello to you,
> It's good to see you today, today.

The first cycle did not include the baby's name, the second did:

> Hello to Maeve, hello to Maeve,
> It's good to see you today, today.
> Hello to Maeve, hello to Maeve,
> It's good to see you today, today.

I used a soft and breathy tone in my singing pitching my voice in my mid to low register. The tune was uncomplicated and moved through simple harmonic sequences. When repeated it brought to my mind the image of a pendulum or perhaps a metronome whose reliable rhythm would aid a sense of relaxation.

The mothers supported their babies on the edges of their laps. I tilted my head down to the babies and sang, looking into their faces. I accompanied my singing on a classical guitar using a finger picking style in 4/4 time. It was a warm and soothing musical environment and each baby, regardless of age or severity of condition, looked into my eyes and held my gaze unwaveringly until the pause after the final chord. Following the 'Hello' song I sang the babies' names over and over improvising with tempo, rhythm and melody. Each of these interactions lasted around 5–7 min during which the remaining group members watched and listened as the music reached into the baby, the mother and the space between them and for that moment held them.

During the period that this holding was happening I too felt held. The light-ness of this feeling was magical and was something I felt long before I ever held my own baby. When I did become a mother I discovered that the feelings evoked in me by music and by my baby were astonishingly similar. At the time as the therapist I was able to observe this lightness and euphoria in myself and attribute it to the music and how it acted as a catalyst in the shift of the mother and baby towards each other. They were jolted out of their apathy and began to be aware of the space between them. The delay in doing this was due, possibly, to the fact that they had not received from each other what they expected in their early encounters. The gleam was absent from the mother's eye and so the baby, not being sufficiently fed by her gaze, was powerless to enter the relating space (Jacoby 1999a). The mother, coping with her baby's disability, was unable to show the feelings of joy in her facial expressions which would allow the baby to start building a healthy sense of themselves and an early understanding of their own actual or potential feeling state (Stern 1995).

This process of transmission of feeling states from mother to baby and baby to mother allows a baby to begin to understand their own reality and experience a sense of self. This attunement (Stern 1995) is of particular interest to me in the context of my thinking about this space between mother and baby and how music might help when the pair faces challenges. The word attunement points immediately to the musical process of moving and changing and adapting musical sounds in order to achieve a workable harmony. It is of course the moving and shifting and adapting of mother and baby to find a similar harmony or attunement throughout their relationship which helps the baby learn about themselves and their identity. 'The affective attunement between the caregiver and the infant serves as the first and most deeply seated influence on its later maturation and development' (Jacoby 1999b p.75)

The types of attunement behaviours that were being displayed between the mothers and babies in the music therapy group seemed to reflect the difficulties in the early relationship resulting in a current block or impasse between the two. My role, I felt, was to facilitate or channel the delivery of music into the pair which could promote effective relating for the time of the session.

One of the pairs with whom I worked included a 12-week-old baby called Maeve. The experience had a lasting impression on me. The mother accessed

Down's syndrome support services very soon after the baby's birth and despite seeming to cynically dismiss the potential of music therapy for herself and her daughter, attended sessions on time and regularly. She enjoyed the support of the other mothers which may have been her motivation for attending in the early sessions. Sessions 1 and 2 were largely introductory and mainly involved helping the mothers feel relaxed enough in the group so that their embarrassment and fear of being sung to was understood and empathized with; the aim being to support them in accessing the full potential of what was being offered. In a discussion about group members' feelings of embarrassment I thought about how these inhibitions about music and the feelings it can evoke in us was mirrored in the vulnerability I saw in these mothers. The classic mechanism for coping with difficult feelings is to try not to feel them at all. So, when music seeps into us and inevitably reaches what it is that we are trying to hide our instinct is to resist. The key was to direct the musical communication to the child who had not learned these inhibitions and who would respond instinctively. This, I predicted, would be the catalyst for the mother's engagement.

So I sang to Maeve:

> Hello to Maeve, hello to Maeve,
> It's good to see you today, today.
> Hello to Maeve, hello to Maeve,
> It's good to see you today, today.

We locked eyes and very soon Maeve's face broke into a radiant smile. The other mothers looked and naturally and instinctively smiled in reply and finally Maeve's mother who was sitting with her child facing away from her, seeing the effect that was spreading throughout the group like candlelight in a cave, looked into her child's face and slowly responded with an almost identical smile followed shortly afterwards by relieved, happy tears. It was the first time Maeve had smiled.

Maeve's mother had an outpouring of emotion that had welled up at the sight of her smiling, happy child. The potential for her child to smile was always there but in the absence of her mother's ability to respond with an encouraging smile it had not yet been seen. The music combined with my very deliberate eye contact and smiling face gave the baby the mirror she needed to unlock her first smile. Not surprisingly the flow of emotion reflected in their expressions to each other thereafter was palpable.

This experience and others like it caused in me a strong emotional response. It was the swell or soar associated with the feeling of real happiness also evoked by playing or listening to certain music. When we listen to music we hear the 'musicalization' of the swell and soar that I refer to. Because the feelings and their musicalization are two sides of the same coin, music can be the earthy element which will act as a catalyst in the healthy attunement between a mother and baby.

So, following the exploration of my combined experiences of motherhood, music and bringing music therapy to mothers and babies, I became more deeply aware of the power and importance of music in the early part of this relationship. Knowing the potential, I decided to try to bring this experience to some of the most vulnerable in our community.

Musical Beginnings at Familiscope

Familiscope is an organization based in a Dublin suburb, Ballyfermot. It is an area of designated social disadvantage which means that children are being raised in communities which are challenged with early school leaving, drug use, criminal behaviour and violence. In the 2006 census data of Ireland 24% of the population of Ballyfermot were documented as lone parents. Faced with these factors these parents are bringing their children up in some of the most unstable and testing environmental circumstances imaginable. Being a parent is one of the greatest challenges facing any person, and becoming a mother in the teenage years brings additional vulnerabilities which the music therapy programme *Musical Beginnings* has sought to address.

A teen mother must contend with a number of added pressures to her experience of mothering. She is in a minority group which in Ireland is not embraced and continues to be responded to with prejudice. She is coping with the pressures of adolescence as well as first time motherhood. She probably lives with her parents and may not have the privacy some older women enjoy in their new parenting role. It is likely that she has not been able to continue her schooling as a result of her pregnancy as some schools in Ireland cannot support teen mothers in the continuation of their education. Due to the pressures of motherhood and the lack of support from schools and society it is unlikely that she will return to school after the birth of her baby. She is likely to be a single parent. Due to her reduced access to education her employment prospects are consequently limited. The support that she receives from the state will not reflect these added pressures and so she may be raising her child on a shoestring leaving no money for her to enjoy her own interests. She may lose touch with her friends and become isolated. While the cohort I have described are at risk for all these added pressures, they are by no means at risk for being inadequate mothers.

However, despite a time of enormous wealth in Ireland, many children are at risk for becoming neglected. Mothers are abandoned by the services that are in place to support and nurture them and the services themselves are often dysfunctional and unhelpful. My experience as a team member at Familiscope is that community services that are available to those that need them are best used by those who are guided in how to access them. In the cases of those that are unable to negotiate their way around complex systems, those systems do not reach out to them and therefore vulnerable mothers and their children are lost.

Familiscope is an organization whose philosophy is to reach out to people and families, bridging the gap between statutory services and those that need them. Those that engage with the service are involved intensively in finding a workable solution to improving their circumstances. The aim is to find the way through the blocks to a place where each individual child, mother, father and family are afforded the opportunity to fulfil their personal potential and build strong relationships.

When I started at Familiscope, I remembered how some of the blocks I saw in my previous professional existence were lifted with the help of music, which acted like a healing balm to support struggling mothers. I saw the potential for music to lend itself to nurturing these young mothers and to support them in building strong relationships with their children in order to go in some way to preventing the kinds of behaviours that are typical in that community. In consideration of this I sought advice in the establishment of a programme from Jane Edwards who had some years before written a successful grant application that supported the formation of an Australian parenting programme called *Sing & Grow* (Abad and Edwards 2004).

Musical Beginnings is a 10-week music therapy programme which uses the music and music therapy elements described in my introduction to promote positive relating between teenage mothers and their new babies. It fits into the framework of Familiscope which is a community-based organization which exists to respond to the needs of the most vulnerable in the community in an area of designated disadvantage in terms of the government's classification of socio-economic indicators. To this end families in which there are children who are at risk for neglect are referred to the service. Following an assessment of each case referred, a care plan is drawn up and carried through in which the child is placed at the centre. The care plan includes a process in which the relevant services are contacted and an exercise in making these services work together efficiently for the benefit of the child and family is executed and monitored. Due to the various areas of neglect; emotional, physical and educational, the interventions are varied. In many cases the teen mother may, herself, be the neglected child who is struggling, in the circumstances of her environment, to raise her child in a positive and nurturing way. It is likely that this is not what her experience as a child with her mother was and so there is an exercise in learning how to be the kind of mother she wants to be.

Musical Beginnings focuses on the development of the mother, the child and the mother and child. The programme recognizes the necessity for the mother to feel good about herself and her potential as a person in order to be the best mother that she can be. The programme focuses on the creative aspects of the mother and child relationship so that a bond is formed which maximizes each individual's scope to feel anchored and secured in this primary relationship. Each individual at their respective points of development can be nourished by the other in this context. This securing and anchoring experience can then release the individuals into a state of being through which their potential can be fulfilled.

Winnicott wrote that it is in playing and only in playing that the individual child or adult is able to be creative and to use the whole personality, and it is only in being creative that the individual discovers the self (Winnicott 1971). This statement reflects the intentions of *Musical Beginnings* which attempts through a specific series of musical interactions and activities to support the global development of the child along with the personal development of the mother.

In the development phase of the programme I spoke to several young women who were either expecting a baby or whose baby had been born. They came to Familiscope's attention through a number of referrers, and came to my notice primarily through the Familiscope Child Welfare Programme; a programme for children who are at risk for neglect due to drug use in the home.

In the development phase of Familiscope[1] it was recommended that a traditional model of delivery of clinical services in which parents and children attend appointments in clinical centres would not be effective. This model results in systems clogged up with waiting lists and eventual loss of the most needy. Arising from this several programmes are being piloted by Familiscope including the delivery of clinical services to children in schools as well as direct sessions and training programmes to teachers. In these programmes techniques are 'given away' to service providers and therefore delivered to children at a very early stage of their development and early education. Built on the principles of early intervention and prevention, the programmes aim to head off potential developmental, behavioural, communication and emotional difficulties. These programmes are ancillary to Familiscope's central programme, the child welfare programme to which I have referred which was born out of reports to the Health Service Executive of chronic cases of neglect.

Familiscope engages with some of the most vulnerable in the community and daily engages with some of the most chronic of neglected persons in the Ballyfermot area and therefore in Ireland. The inherent nature of this cohort is

---

[1] Familiscope was established following the recommendations of the Downes' report prepared by Dr Paul Downes; see www.familiscope.com

that they are made vulnerable by the circumstances of their lives which are largely out of their control. Often their lives include a series of experiences in which they are not protected by their primary carers or formal community services. The carers themselves are likely to have been mistreated in their lives and so the culture and understanding of how they or their children should be cared for is inadequate. This group should be engaged by statutory services but due to a learned cautiousness on their part it can be commonplace for them to avoid these services. This leaves the group in an overwhelmingly vulnerable place. A central focus for Familiscope is to channel its energy into creative and inclusive ways to find those that live in these margins and work with them to return to well being. My aim in developing *Musical Beginnings* for teen mothers and their babies was to use this philosophy and the power of music to ensure that this vulnerable group could experience the kind of bonding described earlier in this account. This bonding or attachment (Bowlby 1969) is what allows the child to develop a healthy sense of self and build self-esteem. It is this healthy self-esteem which motivates persistence at school, in relationships and in the pursuit of potential through the lifespan.

Sarah and Brandon

One of the young women referred to *Musical Beginnings* was Sarah. Her baby, Brandon, was 3 months old when we first spoke. Sarah at 14 years old was a bubbly, smiling girl with a bright, open face. When we spoke I was impressed with her maturity and her articulate expression. She told the difficult story of her life with great empathy for those involved along the way, and without self-pity for the traumatic experiences she had endured in the course of her short life. Recently orphaned, Sarah was deeply committed to the welfare of Brandon and also to the relatives she maintained contact with following the death of her parents.

Sarah did not mention any of her own needs or ambitions. When I broached the subject of the direction she wished her life to take she admitted after some time and with some reservation and embarrassment that she would like to become a nurse. I said that I thought it was a great profession to pursue and asked if she had thought about how she might make a plan to achieve her goal. I offered her the support of the organization in forming this plan and she looked at me quizzically. When I saw this look I suggested that maybe she felt as a mother with a young baby it would be a challenge to organize her time and her baby in order to return to school. She nodded in agreement. I said that I agreed it was difficult and that I too found it hard to balance my own work and interests with my commitment to my children. She said she had not even thought that far ahead. I said such a brave and interesting ambition was indeed within her grasp and that Familiscope would support her in her pursuit of it.

She said that was not the problem. I asked what was. She cast her bright face downwards and said, 'I'm not good enough'. It was a challenge to retain my composure on hearing her say this. To me this girl's achievements were overwhelming. Born into a disadvantaged community where all social expectations would work against her, she had experienced paltry attachment as an infant from a mother who lived in a social exclusion zone in spite of being in one of the wealthiest countries in Europe at that time.

Among this wealth an unhealthy balance was mirrored in the shadow aspect of the community where the collective repressions were being lived out by people with few opportunities, who daily faced mental health challenges, poverty, social and psychological neglect, along with their children. Every one of the stereotypes of these communities was represented in Sarah's family—that is until most of them died. Sarah at the age of 14 was alone. Not long before the death of her mother Sarah's son was born. It was around this time that she came to the notice of Familiscope. In the company of this bright, caring, intelligent, resilient girl I often marvelled at the innate human buoyancy and the personal resources that she drew on for survival.

Sarah was enrolled as a pupil at one of the local Ballyfermot schools. This facility is supportive and welcoming to the pupils who have babies and who wish to re-enter the school system. However, it is often the case that following the birth of their babies girls are more likely to engage in informal education through community services, and like many in her circumstances Sarah was not attending school.

Starting sessions: promoting attendance

Accessing and attending scheduled services is a primary and most challenging goal in working in this area. Familiscope aims to engage the most marginalized and use whatever energy, creativity, time and flexibility that it takes to assist people to access help. By combining my belief in the power of music to support mother and baby attunement with Familiscope's philosophy of maximum support to access by the most vulnerable I aimed to give these mothers and babies the opportunity to nurture the seeds of their early relationships. This opportunity would go in some way to breaking the kinds of cycles, resulting in part from poor early attachment, which lead to early school leaving, challenging behaviour, antisocial behaviour and eventually drug use and other criminal behaviours. My rationale for offering the programme to this group lay in my belief in the importance of early attachment and its power in securing the kind of trust between mothers and babies which would minimize the evolution of these factors.

In the weeks before the first session of the first programme I arranged to meet individually with the mothers who had agreed to attend the programme with their babies. The purpose of this exercise was to reduce the possible barriers of access by the young women to achieve maximum engagement. Some practitioners might argue that an approach like this could sow the seeds of over dependency and disallow the kind of balanced therapeutic relationship that is regarded as necessary for efficacy. However, for those participating in *Musical Beginnings* a whole spectrum of supports and programmes is in place. These are moved forward at a cautious and measured pace aimed at bringing the person to a place where they can manage more independently. If we were to place on our client group the kind of expectation demanded of a more traditional therapeutic relationship we would fail them.

Many of these pre-programme meetings were held in the homes of the mothers and babies. One of these mothers was Christina. The decision to meet in her home followed two attempts to meet in other locations which Christina did not manage to attend. This first meeting went well and I felt it resulted in an increased level of confidence on Christina's part. She agreed to a second meeting, again in her home, and during this meeting we planned for a third. We worked out together that Christina would challenge herself and come to this third meeting in the Familiscope premises. We discussed how important this would be for Christina when the time came to attend *Musical Beginnings*.

I described where Familiscope was located and Christina said she was familiar with the location. We agreed a time and I clarified that Christina's baby Anna would be a delightful and important participant in the meeting. Christina and Anna would come on foot unless it was raining, in which case Familiscope would organize a taxi. Christina asked what would happen when she arrived at Familiscope. I explained that when she arrived at Familiscope's door she would ring the buzzer and I would come down and help her and Anna to come in the door and up the stairs to our Family Room where our meeting would be held. Silence followed. I asked Christina if she felt she could manage this—up to this point in the conversation she had been confident and relaxed. I sat with her and waited. Finally she said that she did not want to ring the buzzer. The prospect of trying to penetrate an anonymous and faceless place was not something she felt confident about. We agreed that when she arrived she would send me a phone message and I would come down and meet her at the door. She was happy with this arrangement. This attention to the step by step process of supporting Christina resulted in her ability to attend the first day.

The programme context and structure

Musical Beginnings weekly sessions were held in a small house in the middle of a large housing estate deemed to house the most vulnerable and at-risk families in Dublin. The idea to hold *Musical Beginnings* within this Family Resource

Centre arose from the knowledge that this place was a gathering point for a wide spectrum of women in the community. At the planning point for the initial programme we realized that while it was desirable to include fathers as well as mothers, it was likely that our first group would be largely women.

The programme structure took its inspiration from the Australian programme *Sing & Grow* (Abad and Edwards 2004). It was 10 weeks in length and each session was 50–60 min in duration. Each session began with a 'Hello' song which was sung to the whole group and then to each individual mother and child using their names. Each mother was encouraged to join in singing to her infant during the 'Hello' song. Every week the women grew in confidence and slowly joined in with the singing. This seemed to mark a shift in each individual towards a stronger sense of togetherness with her child, providing new resources for strengthening their bond. Mothers were encouraged to use these new skills at home.

Following the 'Hello' song nursery songs were sung, many of which included names, body parts and feelings lyrics: 'Heads, Shoulders, Knees and Toes', 'If You're Happy and You Know It', 'The Wheels on the Bus/The Mummys on the Bus/The Babies on the Bus', and other favourites. This was an upbeat section to the session which the mothers and babies seemed to enjoy very much, choosing the verses, singing and moving. It was followed by some instrumental improvisation using individual hand percussion instruments either playing along with a song like 'Twinkle, Twinkle, Little Star' or just freely playing. During this improvisation section we also often used a gathering drum which was useful for call and response sequences and turn taking. The choice of instruments was key to promoting to the parents the idea that the instruments were toys and could be used at home to continue the relationship building during playtime. My hope was that the process of learning the importance of play though music and musical interactions would remain with each mother informing her throughout her relationship with her child of the ongoing need for gentle, empathic interaction and communication. The mothers often commented that these interactions were also easy to replicate at home—a core objective for *Musical Beginnings*.

The final part of the session involved a short relaxation period where mothers were encouraged to place their babies on their laps facing them holding them close to their bodies. I sang soothing songs both improvised and lullabies supporting mums to experience a sense of calm relaxation with their children; an often rare occurrence in the life of a busy parent but nonetheless crucial to a healthy and balanced early relationship. Following this section we often chatted about the importance of the mothers taking time out for themselves. Mothers reported that they thoroughly enjoyed the opportunity to exchange ideas and experiences at this time of ending. The session then ended with a 'Goodbye' song. We would sing goodbye and see you next time to each individual child and mother and then to the group.

Towards the future

I am confident that Sarah and Brandon and Christina and Anna, as well as all the other young mothers and their babies we hope to reach, will have experienced similarly enchanting moments to that of Maeve and her mother. The parts of our lives that many of us take for granted like being on time, having a structure to our day, keeping an appointment or reading a letter are fundamental blocks to some. The isolation and apathy that result from these perceived deficits are blocks and when overcome the same instinct, love, ambition and potential is in place.

Still in its developing days, *Musical Beginnings* is a framework for young women and their babies to come together and meet to share stories of births and weights and feeding and wind, of sleeping and not sleeping. Our desire to exchange notes on these subjects can only be satisfied through conversation with other mothers. The common language and experience of mothers is an essential learning tool. This is the starting point. The therapist must be resilient when faced with the persistent disappointments which occur when group members do not show up following weeks of preparation. The support must resume with the belief that each young woman will appear the next week with her baby in her arms to engage with the musical moments of the session that will remain in their history together forever.

References

Abad, V. and Edwards, J. (2004). Strengthening families: a role for music therapy in contributing to family centred care. *Australian Journal of Music Therapy*, 15, 3–16.

Bowlby, J. (1969). *Attachment and Loss: Volume 1: Attachment.* (London: Hogarth Press)

Jacoby, M. (1999a). *Individuation and Narcissism: the Psychology of Self in Jung and Kohut.* (London: Routledge)

Jacoby, M. (1999b). *Jungian Psychotherapy and Contemporary Infant Research Basic Patterns of Emotional Exchange.* (London: Routledge)

Stern, D.N. (1995). *The Motherhood Constellation.* (New York: Basic Books)

Winnicott, D.W. (1971). *Playing and Reality.* (London: Routledge)

Chapter 9

Extending group music therapy to families in schools: A reflection on practical and professional aspects

Alison Ledger

Parents who initially sat at the back of the room, watching others take turns, play instruments and sing, came to participate through playing instruments and carrying out the actions to songs with their children. Parents who appeared more comfortable in 'rough' play with their children, came to show more affection, through singing gently, swaying their children from side to side, and giving their children hugs and kisses.

Introduction

As the leader of a group music therapy programme for families in Irish schools, I have watched children and their parents enjoying and sharing in music making together. It is rewarding to see parents becoming more involved with their children as sessions progress. At the same time, the work is challenging. Flexibility is needed in order to fit in with long-established school routines and timetables. This chapter explains some of the considerations involved in working within this school-based programme including professional challenges and a range of service delivery issues.

The work described here took place in 2007 when I was employed on an hourly sessional basis for 2 days per week by a charity organization that provides creative arts therapy services to schools in areas referred to as 'disadvantaged'. The mission of this organization is to make emotional supports available to young people in need. By offering creative therapies early in life, the organization's intention is to help young people to realize their full potential.

The support organization had previously identified that families in disadvantaged areas did not have the same access to early childhood music programmes as families in more affluent parts of the city. To address this disparity, parent–child music therapy programmes were introduced to three preschools in disadvantaged areas. These early programmes were highly successful, as demonstrated by other schools contacting the organization to request programmes for their own schools.

When the music therapist who had established this programme left the service, I was recruited to liaise with schools to set up further parent–child programmes. This involved designing, adapting, implementing and evaluating programmes according to the needs in the various school contexts. I was also line manager for a new graduate music therapist employed to deliver some of the groups, and I supervised two music therapy students who led sessions as part of their fieldwork training requirements.

Schools that requested the programme were in areas that continue to receive media attention for feuding, violence, crime, drug and alcohol abuse, young parenthood, and chronic unemployment. Studies of similar communities elsewhere have shown that young children living in these circumstances are at greater risk of developing social, emotional, and academic problems (Leschied et al. 2005; Reid et al. 2007; Smith Battle 2007; Burchinal et al. 2008). It is difficult to separate the effects of individual social risk factors on children. However, there is evidence to support a linked pathway from social disadvantage through parenting quality to children's difficulties in cognitive and language development (Burchinal et al. 2008; Rowe 2008). Some have proposed that economic hardship may lead to parents providing less warmth and necessary stimulation for their children, which in turn may impact on children's skills later in life (Leschied et al. 2005; Burchinal et al. 2008).

Studies have indicated that positive, involved, responsive parenting may buffer the negative impact of risk exposure on children's social skills and academic achievement (Reid et al. 2007; Burchinal et al. 2008). Therefore supportive interventions aimed at improving parents' knowledge, attitude, and skills in relation to their children are recommended (Reid et al. 2007; Rowe, 2008).

Music therapy for parents and their children

The parent–child programme described here was informed by the work of the Australian programme *Sing & Grow* (Abad and Edwards 2004; Abad and Williams 2006; Nicholson et al. 2008). *Sing & Grow* is an early intervention group music therapy programme for families living in communities 'identified as marginal as a result of their socio-economic circumstances' (Abad and Edwards 2004). A range of musical interactions are used to encourage positive parenting behaviours such as smiling, praise, modelling, co-facilitation, and physical affection (Nicholson et al. 2008). Although initially designed for families with children aged birth to 3 years, a large-scale repeated measures evaluation indicated benefits of attending *Sing & Grow* sessions for families with children up to 5 years of age (Nicholson et al. 2008). In this cohort study, an analysis of parents' questionnaire responses and music therapists' ratings revealed significant improvements in parenting behaviours, children's skills, and parents' mental health following participation in the programme (Nicholson et al. 2008).

The parent–child programme that I led was designed for families with children who were attending school, aged from 3 to 6 years. The programme aimed to meet these children's ongoing needs for strengthened family relationships and development of cognitive, language, and social skills. Preschool, junior or senior infant pupils,[1] along with their parents, were invited to attend weekly 1 hour group music sessions in the pupils' class time. In each school, the programme was offered within a particular term and lasted up to 10 weeks.

The programme included children's play songs, songs written by *Sing & Grow* session leaders (Playgroup Association of Queensland 2002), and my own compositions, as well as songs written by the new graduate music therapist and the student music therapists. All of these musical materials aimed to promote positive interactions between family members. Parents and children were encouraged to join together playfully in singing, instrument playing, movement/dancing, and using affectionate touch.

The evaluation of the programme was based on attendance figures, therapists' observations within sessions, verbal and written feedback from teachers, as well as parents' responses on a post-programme survey. Uptake of early childhood interventions is generally reported to be low among families who are marginalized and disadvantaged (Barlow et al. 2005; Nicholson et al. 2008). However, this programme reached 199 families in 2007 and more than half of those who attended were present at six or more sessions.

The programme was evaluated as effective in encouraging positive interactions between family members, developing children's skills and confidence, and promoting supportive relationships between families. Parents who initially sat at the back of the room, watching others take turns, play instruments

---

[1] In other countries, junior infant level is referred to as 'grade one' and senior infant level is referred to as 'grade two'.

and sing, came to participate through playing instruments and carrying out the actions to songs with their children. Parents who appeared more comfortable in 'rough' play with their children, came to show more affection, through singing gently, swaying their children from side to side, and giving their children hugs and kisses. Over the course of each programme, children were observed to increasingly wait their turn to choose and play instruments. Children practised counting and recognized colours in both English and Irish.[2] While singing popular children's songs such as 'Old MacDonald had a Farm', children named animals and suggested animal sounds. Children showed greater confidence as each programme progressed, taking up opportunities to play solos, to be a 'conductor' for the group instrumental play, and to make suggestions for actions or song lyrics. Feedback from teachers and parents indicated that parents had become more involved in the school community through attending the programme.

Practical considerations

This school-based programme enabled access to large numbers of families. In a day's work, I usually attended a single school and worked with up to 30 families. An entire grade level was usually offered the programme, for example all of the preschool classes within one school. As I could remain in the one school seeing groups sequentially, this reduced the amount of time needed for travel, preparing and packing up, and liaising with staff and families.

Teachers as gatekeepers

It was the teacher who initially informed children's parents about the programme and provided me with necessary details about the participants. I therefore met with the classroom teacher prior to the commencement of a programme, to explain the programme aims, to describe what happens in sessions, and to share outcomes from previous programmes. In these meetings, optimal ways of encouraging parents to attend the programme were always discussed. In some schools, it was perceived that a letter to the parents was sufficient, but in others, a short meeting with parents as a group was arranged. In all schools, teachers provided additional information about the programme in informal conversations with parents before and after school.

There were usually 15 or more pupils per class in the schools. These class sizes were too large for successful group therapy. Therapists at *Sing & Grow*, for example, have considered groups of 6–12 parent–child pairs as optimal for

---

2   In Irish primary schools, all children learn Irish as a first or second language (Government of Ireland 1999).

leading and observing individual participants (Nicholson et al. 2008). The teachers' help was therefore sought to divide classes into groups of 10 families or fewer. Separating the classes meant that a proportion of the class needed to be accommodated elsewhere while others were attending music therapy. In schools that were already stretched for space, this was an issue requiring careful negotiation.

In the preschools, it was decided that children would only come to school for the hour long session and then return home afterwards on the day when sessions were held. For junior and senior infant classes, when children were not in a music therapy session they joined in with another class. In one school, teachers expressed concern that this would lead to their own classes becoming unmanageable. In this school then it was agreed not to divide the three senior infant classes. This was only possible because sessions could be co-led by a qualified music therapist and a music therapy student. In this school, introducing a student co-therapist allowed us to include up to 15 families in a session.

Programme participants

Parents were asked to accompany their children to the music therapy sessions for the length of the programme, which was 8–10 weeks depending on the length of the school term. Working parents experienced difficulties in being able to commit to the full programme, as sessions took place during business hours. Sometimes another family member, such as a grandparent, aunt, or older sibling, was asked to attend some or all of the sessions in the place of a parent. It was especially difficult to evaluate families' progress over the course of the programme where the adult attending was not consistent. Furthermore, some children showed disappointment when their primary caregivers did not arrive for the session. For example, one boy declined to join in the session with his 'Nanna', turning away from the group and keeping his arms crossed when his mother did not arrive.

The premise of attachment theory (Bowlby 1969; Ainsworth et al. 1978) is that the child's relationship with his/her primary caregiver is highly important for the child's immediate well being and for their future potential development of emotional capacities (van Ijzendoorn and Schuengel 1999; Shaver and Mikulincer 2005). As this programme aimed to promote positive attachment behaviours between the children and their carers, it is questionable whether children whose primary caregivers were able to attend benefited most from participating in the programme.

Families were not specifically referred to the programme for identified needs as in other parent–child music therapy programmes (Oldfield et al. 2003; Abad and Edwards 2004; Molyneux 2005). Rather, participants were selected because of their attendance at a particular school, and the evident social deprivation of the environs. Needs were therefore determined by the therapists in observing families' interactions within sessions. Some parents were observed to have difficulties interacting with their children. These parents overlooked their children's needs for encouragement and assistance, or handled their children in a forceful manner when requesting them to participate. Other parents appeared to have close affectionate relationships with their children, and easily interacted through shared singing, instrument play, laughing, and affectionate touch. Some of the children showed attention, behavioural, and/or language difficulties for their age, but the majority appeared to be developing healthily for their respective ages.

In working to identify and address the needs of so many families, there were instances when I felt that some families' unique needs may not have been met. At the same time, the inclusion of families who related well could also be viewed positively, as confident and responsive parents were helpful models for other parents. They showed enthusiasm for the programme and demonstrated ways of participating and interacting positively and gently with their children. Furthermore, the inclusion of a range of families reinforces growing discourse that *all* children should have access to musical experiences, regardless of socioeconomic status (Mackenzie and Hamlett 2005; Young 2007). By including all children within a year level, music therapists may play an important role in promoting music making to all families as a means to build successful rapport and relating.

Therapy spaces

In most schools, sessions took place in the children's classrooms. These rooms were chosen as they were available and familiar to children and their parents. The children's classrooms were busy, colourful spaces, filled with posters, children's artwork, toys, books, puzzles, and games. There were times when these features appeared to distract families from the therapy work. Sometimes children left the group to play elsewhere in the room instead of joining their parents in the session. There were also moments when sessions were interrupted by other teachers or students entering the classroom.

In two schools, sessions took place in a separate vacant room in the school. These seemed to be more appropriate spaces for therapeutic work as there were fewer distractions and interruptions. Some simple steps did seem to help minimize disruptions. For example, toys could be tidied before the start of a session, or a 'do not disturb' sign could be placed on the classroom door. It took time to develop strategies that worked in each school and inevitably some days the programme staff arrived to find that a different activity had been planned in the usual therapy space. Flexibility and persistence were required to establish the best possible spaces for therapy sessions.

Emergent professional issues
Roles and responsibilities

Prior to this programme, I had worked mostly within multidisciplinary health-care teams. This was the first time in my career as a music therapist that I worked in schools. My co-workers were no longer other allied health professionals, but instead teachers. Classroom teachers assisted with the set-up of programmes and attended the group music therapy sessions. I was not aware of any other therapists working so closely with the teachers in the schools. The respective roles and responsibilities of the teacher and the therapist therefore developed over time, as experience and knowledge of the context and each other grew.

In many of the schools, teachers' involvement in sessions contributed to the success of the programme. By participating in sessions, teachers provided excellent models for the parents and children and communicated that the programme was important and beneficial to them.

The inclusion of teachers in the sessions could be likened to co-leadership arrangements, in which two leaders have separate roles (Fearn and O'Connor 2003). When a teacher was enthusiastic and involved, parents and children appeared motivated to attend and participate. Teachers often responded to my encouragement to participate actively in sessions, and also used their own initiative to assist me in leading the sessions. For example, teachers played an important role when parents brought younger siblings to the sessions. Teachers offered to hold these younger children, or sometimes set up a separate area with a quiet activity for them. This allowed parents to focus their attention on the child who was in the class.

At other times, the presence of teachers appeared to distract participating families. Although asked to sit within the group, some teachers moved away to complete other tasks in the classroom. A memorable example was when a teacher and a classroom assistant were making Easter decorations at the side of the therapist in the classroom. The children kept looking over to them, talking excitedly about the eggs and 'bunnies', rather than engaging in the therapy group.

In some sessions, a teacher took on the responsibility of disciplining children. This occurred when a child was not following directions, did not wait his/her turn, moved to take another child's instrument, or was causing a safety risk, such as waving a drum stick in the air, or running around the group.

In the disciplining of children in this context it was unclear whether the teachers relieved parents of this responsibility. Some parents never stepped in to intervene, even when their children were causing considerable disruption to a session. In these cases, did teachers provide examples of how these parents could discipline their children? Or did teachers minimize opportunities for parents to practise skills? Would parents have intervened if a teacher was not present? In retrospect, it would have been advantageous to discuss disciplining roles with teachers and parents before the start of each programme and perhaps establish some simple ground rules.

At times there seemed to be 'too many cooks' in the room. Sometimes this meant that the teacher led the group in a direction that was different to the one I had intended. I remember a time when I was attempting to bring a high-energy session to a close, so as to prepare participants for moving on to the next part of the session. I began to play quieter and slowed down the tempo of the music. However, the classroom teacher continued to encourage the participants to sing loudly and to move energetically to the music. This made it difficult for me to achieve my aim of calming participants and instead the group ended 'on a high'.

Of course these teachers had pre-established leadership roles in working with the children and their parents prior to the programme. To implement the programme successfully, the therapist needed to develop a leadership presence. It was inevitable that power negotiation was needed. If teachers are to be included in sessions, it can be worthwhile to discuss in detail each person's roles and responsibilities within the group. Inviting constructive feedback from teachers can also maximize benefits for families and avoid possible misunderstandings and resentments.

Classroom teachers' assistance in setting up the programme was highly valued. However, by keeping the teacher as the main contact person for families, I felt that therapists' opportunities to get to know parents were limited. I interacted with parents musically throughout sessions, but rarely had a chance to talk with them outside sessions. I only attended each school on a weekly basis and often sessions were conducted straight after one another. This restricted the amount of time available for learning parents' names and for listening to individual concerns about their children and family relationships. I expect that parents would gain more from the programme if they were to have one to one contact with the therapist before or after sessions.

Teachers provided helpful information regarding families' needs, including information about physical disabilities, communication disorders, and relationship difficulties at home. However, this did not replace the input of a team highly skilled in the identification and treatment of such difficulties. Had a psychologist, social worker, or other allied health professional been available, I could have sought their advice on ways of interacting with some participants. It was difficult to leave a school at the end of a programme when families had presented with difficulties and there was no immediate qualified personnel to whom they could be referred.

On reflection I would have liked to have found a way to discover more about parents' perceptions of the role of the teacher within the programme. It is reasonable to expect that returning to the classroom reminded parents of their own schooling experiences, particularly as some of the parents had attended the same school that their children were now attending, and their experiences may or may not have been positive. I explored various questions to help give consideration to this issue. Did parents expect to be evaluated by the teacher? Did parents fear they would 'get in trouble' from the teacher if they were not 'good enough'? Could these concerns have influenced their levels of participation? I did not ask the parents directly and so am unsure of the answers to these questions. However, I always observed teachers to be encouraging towards parents.

Music therapy or 'Music for Fun'

In imparting information to parents about the programme, teachers appeared uncomfortable using the word 'therapy'. I was told that there was considerable stigma attached to the word and that 'if we call it therapy, people won't come'. In some schools, teachers referred to the programme as 'music for fun and learning' instead of 'music therapy' in their letters to parents. One teacher wished to reassure parents that 'you don't have to participate' in her letter to parents. As the programme was designed in order that parents would join in the music making with their children, I negotiated a rewording of the letter to include singing, instrument playing, moving, and relaxing to music. The suggestion that parents should play a passive role in sessions was removed.

While I wanted as many parents as possible to attend, I felt that they were entitled to know that they would be receiving 'music therapy'. I considered it my ethical responsibility to provide adequate information to families about myself and the programme. I wanted to be honest and clear and for parents to have some understanding of what they were agreeing to attend. I did not want to imply that all families were experiencing difficulties, but at the same time I wanted families to use the programme to work on their relationships. If parents did not know what the programme was addressing, how could they know how to participate and improve their skills? I therefore made sure to introduce myself as a 'music therapist' in my initial sessions with families. I stated that the weekly 1 hour session was a time for parents to spend some 'quality time' with their children. I also explained that parents could help their children by singing and assisting them to carry out the actions to songs, to play instruments, and to move to music. The programme aims were restated periodically over the 8–10 weeks.

A fundamental aspect of many music therapy programmes is that clients are given choice over their participation (Dileo 2000; Daveson 2001). As teachers were encouraged to present the programme as one that parents or children's nominated guardians were required to attend, it is reasonable to expect that parents viewed the programme as compulsory. Conducting the programme in schools potentially limited the families' rights to choose whether or not to attend. An alternative view is that by likening the programme to a compulsory learning opportunity such as a class field trip, teachers ensured greater attendance to the initial session than would have been realized had the programme been presented as optional. When parents attended the first session and had then seen the programme for themselves, it was presumed they could make an informed decision as to whether or not to continue attending.

Reaching families at risk is often regarded as challenging (Barlow et al. 2005; Nicholson et al. 2008) and it is easy to assume that families will not understand, do not want to change, or will not want to come. Research has indicated that some parents misperceive the aims of an early intervention service or the type of support being offered (Barlow et al. 2005). However, in my experience parents easily saw the benefits of a programme for themselves. When asked in a post-programme survey what they liked best about the programme, parents regularly referred to the interaction or involvement with their children; for example, 'contact with the child', 'one to one with my child'. This suggests that parents do value opportunities to strengthen relationships with their children and may attend programmes designed to assist them in this regard. I feel that it is possible to afford parents greater responsibility over their participation and progress in the programme, as advocated by other music therapists (Daveson 2001; Barlow et al. 2005; Rolvsjord 2006). Additionally, parents should be asked for their perceptions regarding their families' needs (Barlow et al. 2005).

Attendance is an aspect which we can readily observe, quantify, and report to management and funding bodies. Attendance figures can also be used to show that levels of parent satisfaction and retention are greater than that expected for traditional parenting programmes and that money given to music therapy programmes is well spent (Abad and Williams 2006; Nicholson et al. 2008). However, I wonder whether families' progress over the course of a programme is more important, even if the number of families who attend is small.

Issues of inclusion and exclusion

There were times when a parent brought a child to school but did not join his/her child for the music therapy session. Whether children should be able to attend sessions unaccompanied was a challenging issue. On principle, I proposed that children should not attend alone when the programme aimed to strengthen family relationships. Most of the musical opportunities in the sessions required two people, a child and a parent, and children often needed adult assistance to join in.

Other adults who were present could offer help to a child, but could not replace the role of a parent. Consideration of possible negative ramifications for a child who realizes that everyone except him/herself has the support of a family member is needed. It was a difficult situation to manage when no guardian arrived and a child was subsequently unable to join the group. With experience, I learned to discuss with teachers the benefits and disadvantages of including unaccompanied children in sessions. Decisions were made as to how best to address this situation, but these decisions rarely remained consistent.

In a school where it was decided to exclude children who were not accompanied, a junior infant student appeared angry and aggressive when asked to leave and go to another classroom. He ran away outside and swore at his teacher when she attempted to encourage him to return inside the school. This led his teacher and I to rethink whether he should be included in sessions, as perhaps it was most important for him to remain with his classmates. In another school, it was decided that all children should be included in sessions, regardless of whether they were accompanied by a parent or guardian. A senior infant student then showed her disappointment that her mother did not arrive. She sat in the group with her arms folded and eyes cast downward. She declined all offers of help from the adults present, before spinning herself around in the centre of the group, showing her feelings of abandonment. The teachers and I were concerned that sessions without her parent may have been detrimental to this student. Without her mother in the sessions, the student may have felt unattended to, unsupported, maybe even unloved.

Ultimately it was difficult to set concrete rules about the inclusion of unaccompanied children. Children's reactions to being unaccompanied could be difficult to predict and often changed from week to week. This emphasizes a need to remain flexible in this work, to continually monitor children's responses, and to make decisions accordingly.

Structure and expression

In some ways, the school setting was ideal for contributing to the children's development. In designing the music therapy programme, the therapists were able to work closely with the teachers to include concepts that children were already learning in school; for example, colours, numbers, and Irish words. The children were already familiar with being asked to sit together in a group, to listen to others, to follow directions, and to wait their turns within the classroom environment. This meant that it was less challenging for the therapists to lead the music therapy groups and to build upon these important social skills. It is also possible that similarities between the rules of the classroom and the routines of the therapy group may have enabled transfer of skills across the two settings.

From a different perspective, the school environment is one that has traditionally focused more on the development of concepts and skills than the development of emotional expression. Even in the early school years, there continues to be a strong emphasis on the rudiments of communication, literacy, and numeracy. The importance of self-expression and creativity is only now being emphasized in education policies (Young 2007). For this reason, I felt unable to address parenting issues to the extent that may have been possible in a different setting. If a parent was seen to be missing opportunities to assist or share in music making with his/her child, then further participation was encouraged through modelling, verbal directions, or praise. This was observed to be successful in increasing parents' participation in sessions. However, I wondered whether more could be done to motivate parents to improve their parenting skills, to help parents to identify their own children's needs, and to offer parents further ways of interacting with their children. As the programme took place in schools, the focus seemed to be more on developing the children's skills than on improving the skills of the parents. This was evident in one parent's comment on the post-programme survey, 'I think the children really enjoyed it, but I'm not sure if there was a real need for the parents to attend also'. This indicated that more efforts need to be taken to promote the programme as one that helps parents to develop their skills too.

Were changes lasting?

It is challenging to consider whether a 10-week school-based programme was sufficient to achieve lasting change for participating families. The degree to which positive family interactions were maintained was evaluated through the use of a post-programme survey. After the final sessions, parents or other participating family members rated aspects of the sessions on a scale from 1 (not at all) to 5 (very much) and answered closed and open-ended questions about their experiences. While almost all agreed that their families had enjoyed the programme, responses were more varied on survey items pertaining to the degree of change outside of sessions. Some respondents gave neutral or negative responses to the statement 'The music sessions helped me get to know my child even better'. Not all guardians agreed that they had 'used more music at home' since coming to the sessions. It was not clear whether the programme was unsuccessful in achieving lasting change for these families, or whether these respondents considered that they already had strong bonds with their children and sang and played at home prior to attending the programme.

To assist families to maintain improvements in their relationships, a follow-up programme was introduced with the start of a new school year (at the end of 2007). This shorter 6-week programme, including new songs and musical play, was offered to families who had participated in the programme previously. Early reports from the participating music therapist, teachers, and families indicated that the follow-up programme was effective in promoting the gains achieved in the previous year.

Conclusion

A range of practical and professional issues were encountered in implementing this parent–child music therapy programme in schools. Although challenging, this experience provided me with a valuable opportunity to develop and reflect upon my roles and responsibilities as a music therapist in this context. Flexibility and compromise were required, in order to implement programmes that met the needs of participating schools and groups of families.

In spite of the challenges described, the development of a school-based programme was a novel and important way to offer support to and find ways to connect with potentially vulnerable families. Music therapists are encouraged to build on this work, in order to continue to meet children's ongoing needs for strengthened family relationships.

References

Abad, V., and Edwards, J. (2004). Strengthening families: a role for music therapy in contributing to family centred care. *The Australian Journal of Music Therapy*, 15, 3–17.

Abad, V., and Williams, K. (2006). Early intervention music therapy for adolescent mothers and their children. *British Journal of Music Therapy*, 20, 31–38.

Ainsworth, M.D.S., Blehar, M.C., Waters, E., and Wall, S. (1978). *Patterns of Attachment: a Study of the Strange Situation*. (Hillsdale, NJ: Erlbaum)

Barlow, J., Kirkpatrick, S., Stewart-Brown, S., and Davis, H. (2005). Hard-to-reach or out of reach? Reasons why women refuse to take part in early interventions. *Children and Society*, 19, 199–210.

Bowlby, J. (1969). *Attachment and Loss: Volume 1: Attachment.* (London: Hogarth)

Burchinal, M., Vernon-Feagans, L., Cox, M., and Key Family Life Project Investigators. (2008). Cumulative social risk, parenting, and infant development in rural low-income communities. *Parenting Science and Practice*, 8, 41–69.

Daveson, B.A. (2001). Empowerment: an intrinsic process and consequence of music therapy practice. *The Australian Journal of Music Therapy*, 12, 29–38.

Dileo, C. (2000). Clients' rights and therapists' responsibilities. In C. Dileo (ed.) *Ethical Thinking in Music Therapy*, pp. 75–95. (Cherry Hill, NJ: Jeffrey Books)

Fearn, M.C., and O'Connor, R. (2003). The whole is greater than the sum of its parts: experiences of co-working as music therapists. *British Journal of Music Therapy*, 17, 67–75.

Government of Ireland (1999). *Primary School Curriculum*. (Dublin: Government Stationery Office)

Leschied, A.W., Chiodo, D., Whitehead, P.C., and Hurley, D. (2005). The relationship between maternal depression and child outcomes in a child welfare sample: implications for treatment and policy. *Child and Family Social Work*, 10, 281–291.

Mackenzie, J., and Hamlett, K. (2005). The Music Together program: addressing the needs of 'well' families with young children. *The Australian Journal of Music Therapy*, 16, 43–59.

Molyneux, C. (2005). Music therapy as a short-term intervention with individuals and families in a child and adolescent mental health service. *British Journal of Music Therapy*, 19, 59–66.

Nicholson, J.M., Berthelsen, D., Abad, V., Williams, K., and Bradley, J. (2008). Impact of music therapy to promote positive parenting and child development. *Journal of Health Psychology*, 13, 226–238.

Oldfield, A., Adams, M., and Bunce, L. (2003). An investigation into short-term music therapy with mothers and young children. *British Journal of Music Therapy*, 17, 26–45.

Playgroup Association of Queensland. (2002). *Sing & Grow Together* [CD]. (Brisbane: Playgroup Association of Queensland)

Reid, M.J., Webster-Stratton, C., and Hammond, M. (2007). Enhancing a classroom social competence and problem-solving curriculum by offering parent training to families of moderate- to high-risk elementary school children. *Journal of Clinical Child and Adolescent Psychology*, 36, 605–620.

Rolvsjord, R. (2006). A discussion on music and power-relations in music therapy. *British Journal of Music Therapy*, 20, 5–12.

Rowe, M.L. (2008). Child-directed speech: relation to socioeconomic status, knowledge of child development and child vocabulary skill. *Journal of Child Language*, 35, 185–205.

Shaver, P.R., and Mikulincer, M. (2005). Attachment theory and research: resurrection of the psychodynamic approach to personality. *Journal of Research in Personality*, 39, 22–45.

Smith Battle, L. (2007). Legacies of advantage and disadvantage: the case of teen mothers. *Public Health Nursing*, 24, 409–420.

Van Ijzendoorn, M.H., and Schuengel, C. (1999). The development of attachment relationships. In D. Messer, and S. Millar (eds) *Exploring Developmental Psychology*, pp. 82–103. (London: Arnold)

Young, S. (2007). Early childhood music education in England: changes, choices, and challenges. *Arts Education Policy Review*, 109, 19–26.

Chapter 10

Music therapy to support mothers who have experienced abuse in childhood

Toni Day and Helen Bruderer

For every day my body aches
Reliving this life of pain
The dark memories scattered in my head have driven
me insane
The memories I have of you mostly occurred on dark
nights
For these were the scariest 'cause there were no lights
The dark of night holds the key to her fright
Love her, don't hurt her and
never turn out the light.
© A.J. 2001

Introduction

Music therapy can offer support to women who have experienced childhood abuse. A project providing 12 weekly sessions for 20 women in three different groups found that the process of writing songs and then recording and performing these songs contributed to a sense of pride and achievement for participants. For some of the women this process was experienced as providing closure on their childhood experiences.

This programme was facilitated by a social worker and music therapist. It was designed to enable the women participants to explore and resolve their experiences so that they were able to parent more effectively and safely. The women participants had experienced childhood physical, emotional and sexual abuse and were identified as 'at risk' of continuing the cycle of abuse with their own children. Therefore the facilitators worked within a therapeutic as well as educative approach to parenting support.

The use of music within this programme, and in particular song writing, was an innovative addition to a creative and innovative model of parenting education. By addressing the needs of these parents regarding their abusive childhood experiences, their ongoing attachments with their own children was able to be strengthened.

Child abuse and parenting

Courtois (2000) has described child abuse as a 'form of traumatic stress that holds an inordinately high potential to impact and to traumatise both the child victim in its immediate aftermath and the adult survivor across the life span' (p. xv). Child abuse is associated with multiple risk factors such as low socio-economic status, family disruption, domestic violence, and substance abuse (Australian Institute of Health and Welfare 2006). The more frequent, the more prolonged and the more serious the abuse or neglect, the more damaging it will be for the child (NSW Commission for Children and Young People 2000). Regardless of the type of abuse experienced during childhood, adult survivors may experience increased rates of mental health problems (Fergusson et al. 2008), sexual difficulties, decreased self-esteem, and interpersonal problems (O'Brien 1991; Mullen et al. 1996). Continued abuse may lead to problems with sexuality, including ongoing questions about gender identity, types of sexual expression or preference (Maltz and Holman 1987). As Hall (2008) has noted:

> . . . clinical experience suggests that men and women who were sexually abused in childhood often feel like 'damaged goods,' especially when it comes to their sexuality. Feeling obliged to comply with a model of 'normal' sexual functioning then produces renewed anxiety and shame in addition to confusion about what is 'normal'. (Hall 2008 p. 547)

Abuse survivors may be left with a variety of mixed emotions, including anger, grief, fear, powerlessness, and depression. They can lose their sense of self and becoming numb may be the only way they can exist in an unsafe environment (Rogers 2003). Most children abused in their childhood leave their secrets intact until they reach adulthood (Herman 1997). A Swedish study of adolescents that included 2324 girls and 2015 boys showed that some kind of sexual abuse had occurred for more than 23% of the males and 65% of the female respondents. Most teenagers in the study who indicated they had reported the sexual abuse had disclosed the information to a peer rather than to an adult or health professional. This indicates that the problems related to the high incidence and prevalence of abuse in childhood continue to remain 'hidden' from adult society (Priebe and Svedin 2008).

There is an increasing realization that parents abused during their own childhoods can face difficulties in parenting (Haapasalo and Aaltonen 1999). In particular, it is noted that increased permissive practices, and lack of authoritarian or boundary setting parenting can occur (Ruscio 2001). Survivors of childhood sexual abuse (CSA) may have difficulty coping effectively with the emotional demands involved in child rearing (DiLillo et al. 2000). It is also recognized in trying to understand the effects of childhood sexual abuse that 'the association between CSA and parenting outcomes may not always be simple or direct. Parenting is a complex, multidimensional process that is vulnerable to a variety of influences such as socioeconomic status, marital factors and stress' (Schuetze and Das Eiden 2005 p. 646).

Aversive childhood experiences may predispose parents to become depressed and stressed, consequently decreasing the quality of their interaction with their child (Ethier et al. 1995). Mothers who were abused as children and were also neglecting or abusing their own children, have been reported to have high stress levels, and be living in disruptive and unstable home environments (Ethier et al. 1995).

Appropriate expression of anger is one of the more common emotional difficulties experienced by those with a history of childhood sexual abuse (Scott and O'Neil 1996). Both practice and research wisdom point to the unmet basic emotional needs of parents as a crucial factor in the quality of interactions between parents and children.

Parenting education programmes

Most parents undertake the role of parenting with little preparation except their own experiences as a child. Their parenting is also shaped by their own personality, the characteristics of the child and their family, and wider social support networks (Bowes 2000). For parents whose original home was one where they were neglected or abused, new information is needed to assist them to parent more effectively than they were parented (Bowes 2000). Parenting education programmes have been demonstrated to assist both the parent and their children, with positive effects maintained at follow-up (Pinquart and Teubert 2010).

Within the child abuse prevention literature there continues to be a focus on family support programmes having two major roles. The first is to provide counselling and support, which may incorporate respite care or a home visiting service to families who are defined as 'at risk' of maltreating their child and are socially isolated. Secondly, these programmes aim to enhance parenting skills by providing parenting education (Poole and Tomison 2000). Child development information and parenting advice are included in most parent education programmes (Bowes 2000). This information is seen as crucial in preventing child abuse and neglect and to help parents give their children a strong emotional, social and intellectual start to their lives.

Ideal characteristics of parent education and family support services for vulnerable and 'at-risk' families

Parenting and support programmes for vulnerable parents ideally need to be flexible, holistic and therapeutic. They need to address issues that impact on both the individual and the family such as anger, lack of trust, low self-esteem, lack of self-care and self-awareness.

Dale et al. (1989) observed that parents who have physically harmed their children have invariably experienced 'deprived and disturbed childhoods with high levels of violence, alcoholism and neglect in their families of origin' (p. 185), and as a result of this, the 'self-protective response of denial of one's own feelings and suppression of anger is learned' from which 'the seeds of explosive anger are sown' (Dale et al. 1989 p.186). O'Brien (1991) has stated 'that it is essential to first work therapeutically with those parents to heal the unresolved hurt and anger so that it does not remain as an ever ready time bomb, waiting to be triggered by the day to day crises that occur in caring for children' (p. 20). Parenting support and education programmes therefore need to offer supportive responses to participants so that the hurt from child-hood abuse experiences can begin to be acknowledged and resolved with the ultimate goal of supporting parents to parent effectively and safely.

Music therapy intervention within parenting programmes

Music therapy support for survivors of childhood abuse has been described by music therapy clinicians and researchers (Cassity and Theobold 1990; Clendenon-Wallen, 1991; Montello 1999; Whipple and Lindsey 1999; Rogers 2003; Amir 2004; Austin 2006). However, limited literature has outlined the use of music therapy techniques within parenting programmes that address needs of parents' experiences of childhood abuse. Lyons (2000) described the incorporation of music techniques within a social group with mothers and babies. These mothers were marginalized from mainstream society and experiencing difficulties relating to their own childhood trauma, domestic violence, substance abuse, and mental health problems. The main focus of this work was to foster both parent–child interaction and parents' mutual aid (Lyons 2000).

Oldfield and Bunce (2001) have described music therapy work that is designed to encourage a deeper level of attachment and enhance relationships between parents and young children through structured, non-verbal musical activities. Similarly the Australian project *Sing & Grow* (Abad and Edwards 2004; Nicholson et al. 2008) is an early intervention group-based music therapy programme that is designed to enhance attachment between vulnerable parents and infants.

Therapeutic outcomes of song writing

The therapeutic effect of writing a song within therapy sessions is brought about through the client's creation, performance and/or recording of his or her own song (Baker and Wigram 2005). Edgerton (1990) stated that authors and researchers describe song writing as an effective music therapy technique in achieving goals such as group cohesiveness, increasing self-expression and self-esteem, improving interpersonal communication, recovering repressed material and enhancing insight into personal issues.

Song writing is well suited to the group setting as it provides groups with opportunities to share and affirm feelings, receive approval from peers, and also express feelings in a confidential and safe environment (MacIntosh 2003). Song writing has been used elsewhere to increase appropriate expression of anger; to explore personal boundaries, trust and sexuality; and to develop problem-solving skills (Clenendon-Wallen 1991). The authors have elsewhere reported the processes of song writing to support participants in a parenting group for survivors of sexual abuse in childhood (Bruderer 2007; Day 2007).

A human rights framework

This parenting project was informed by the principles of human rights underpinned by the principles of social justice (Chenoweth and McAuliffe 2005). The principle of human rights particularly pertinent to this project is the 'first generation of rights', often referred to as civil and political rights. These are regarded as being fundamental to a fair and effective democracy and civil society. This includes the right to be treated with dignity and to be free from discrimination, intimidation or torture (Chenoweth and McAuliffe 2005).

The social work profession understands social justice to encompass all of the following; the satisfaction of basic human needs; the equitable distribution of resources to meet these needs; fair access to public services and benefits to achieve human potential; recognition of individual and community rights and duties; equal treatment and protection under the law; social development and environmental management in the interests of human welfare (Australian Association of Social Workers 2002).

The programme also employed many of the principles of the 'strengths perspective framework' (Saleeby 1997). Underpinning the strengths perspective is the belief that every individual, group, family and community has strengths. The lexicon of this perspective is empowerment, membership, resilience, healing and wholeness (Saleebey 1997). Anderson (1997) has stated,' . . . when we focus on strengths, we do not overlook real limitation and pathology. We recognise untapped reserves of energy, integrity, courage, fortitude and desire for change' (p. 17).

Additionally, the programme was informed from feminist and narrative theories (White and Denborough 1998; Hadley 2006). The feminist principles supporting the framework of the project included empowerment, inclusiveness, consciousness-raising, and the breaking down of power dichotomies (Payne 1994). Using a narrative approach was intended to enable participants to go beyond the oppression of the dominant stories about themselves, and begin to have access to new, empowering stories about their own resourcefulness and survival (White and Denborough 1998).

Respectful conflict resolution was also an important aspect of this project. As O'Brien (1991) has noted,

> The process of openly resolving conflict in a group is something entirely new for these parents. Sometimes parents have difficulty expressing themselves but usually this changes with increasing confidence. More commonly, parents go off on tangents when articulating and this makes it very hard for others in the group to follow or understand the whole nature of what is being described. (O'Brien 1991 p. 22)

Music therapy group work for mothers who have experienced abuse in childhood

Three parent support groups that used music therapy techniques were developed following on from a pilot project successfully conducted in 1998. The pilot had used song writing to address issues around parenting and domestic violence with 12 women identified as being 'at risk' of harm, or who had previously harmed their children. All but one of these parents identified that they had experienced abuse in their childhood that had never been addressed.

Following a successful grant application to the Department of Families and Community Services in Australia, three groups were held over a 1-year period, each comprising 12 workshop style sessions. The primary objectives of the project included: (a) supporting the participants to break the intergenerational cycle of abuse through developing or enhancing their attachment with their children/newborn; (b) developing or enhancing positive communication with their children thereby reducing the risk of harm to the children; (c) supporting the parents not only to parent safely but to begin to enjoy their parenting role and their children: and (d) allowing participants to express themselves by sharing their stories and having their feelings validated, in order to develop and/or enhance their emotional well-being.

The programme culminated in the recording of the women's song creations. The workshops were held in community settings which were easy to access via public transport. The workshops were provided free of costs to participants and childcare and refreshments were provided. Thus, the mothers did not have to attend to their children during the time of the workshops.

A portable CD player and a range of percussion instruments were available for the groups each week along with a guitar and keyboard. The duration of the workshops was usually 2 hours although often this time was extended to provide further individual support for group members as required. The facilitators also offered ongoing support after the formal group contact had finished each day as needed.

The leaders employed an educative and therapeutic approach using the group process and incorporating principles from the disciplines of social work and music therapy. The main music therapy technique used in this project was song writing. Initially instrumental improvisation was offered but participants indicated some resistance. They showed fearful expressions and avoided picking up an instrument when offered the opportunity. Comments directed towards the music therapy facilitator such as 'That's what you are here for Toni' indicated some of the group members' reluctant feelings about contributing to this type of music making.

Song listening therefore became an important part of the group process and was used to initiate discussion and interaction. Participants were encouraged at the commencement of the workshops to bring in some of their own music to share with group members. This approach assisted participants to reveal ideas and thoughts that needed to be examined and discussed, as well as encouraging participants to access feelings that needed to be expressed and shared. This became a starting place for the discussion of more personal issues.

Saleebey (1997) stated that one of the characteristics of being oppressed is having one's stories buried beneath the landslide of stereotype and ignorance. A story told and appreciated offers affirmation for a person, family, or culture (Saleebey 1997). The facilitators became aware that the workshop context was the first time the majority of these women could tell their story and be heard.

The project participants

Twenty women attended the project. The decision to only include women was based on previous experience in the field where women had described not feeling comfortable talking about their abuse with other male participants or facilitators. The programme was designed to offer assistance with parenting issues within a family support programme. Therefore, only women with children, and/or women who were pregnant were included. As the project aimed to support women abuse survivors, all participants had experienced abuse in childhood.

Information about the women was gathered through a voluntary initial intake survey which also gathered basic demographic s. Of the participants, fourteen had experienced all forms of abuse including physical, sexual, emotional/ psychological and neglect; seventeen had experienced sexual abuse; seventeen had experienced physical abuse; and nineteen had experienced emotional and psychological abuse. All participants indicated that they had first experienced this abuse under the age of 8 years. Nineteen of the twenty participants were parents of infants and/or young children. Two of the participants were pregnant, one with her first child. Some of the participants were self-referred while others attended after being referred through agencies such as sexual assault services, the Social Work Department at the Royal Women's Hospital in Brisbane, domestic violence organizations, refuges and the Parent Aide Unit, Royal Children's Hospital, Brisbane.

Groups were closed[1] and intentionally small in number. Two of the groups had eight members, and one had four. Weekly attendance was encouraged to allow for consistent group membership. This was considered important due to the sensitive nature of the issues being explored and the need to establish an environment of safety and trust.

Although their childhood experiences had obviously affected them in varying ways, the women shared the common desire to stop the intergenerational cycle of child abuse and learn ways to parent more safely. They also shared the desire for their stories to be heard. The voices of women who come from backgrounds of this kind are very rarely sought or heard.

The group process: early, middle and termination

Although there were differences experienced within each programme, the process for each group followed a similar pattern that involved three main stages, early, middle and termination (Glassman et al. 1990).

---

[1] This means that the people who would attend were agreed in advance and no new members could join once the programme had started. This is a common approach in group work to support feelings of security and safety among group members.

Early stages of the group

Weeks 1–4 were the more uncomfortable, reflecting the anxiety and tension of this early phase of group development. Members' attendance and participation was irregular. O'Brien (1991) has stated that 'attendances are likely to be inconsistent until the parent trusts the whole group and feels that she belongs in that group' (p. 21). During this stage group members had to build trust. This was particularly challenging because of the needs and prior experience of the women. Joining exercises and warm up activities were used to assist participants to get to know each other and encourage participation. On Day 1 of the three groups, we began with the streamer exercise where all members were asked to individually speak of the need or issue that had brought them to group. They then connected with another member of their choice by throwing them a streamer that then gave that member the opportunity to speak. By the end of the exercise all members were connected by the streamer giving a spider web effect symbolic of the communication and relationship web that would unfold over the coming weeks.

During this early phase 'strength cards'[2] that included a word or phrase of encouragement were used to prompt discussion and identify personal and parenting strengths. For most of the women this was a new concept. Participants reported negative perceptions about themselves and their parenting abilities. Focusing on strengths was intended to assist the women to discover self-worth and self-identity in their abilities to survive (Blundo 2001).

Music listening was also used at this stage to gain further understanding of the participants. In Week 1, the facilitators chose songs relevant to the reason for the group and spoke about their choice. From Week 2 onwards participants selected and brought their significant songs to the group. On occasions we had to source the requested CD as participants had no access to it. Participants spoke about the songs and their relevance to their lives. Other participants were asked to listen and at times this was quite difficult for some group members especially if it was a style of music they disliked. This technique gave much insight into the group members as well as an opportunity to begin to open up to the group slowly and to experience being heard within the group.

As facilitators, we were more actively involved in Weeks 1–4 and especially the first 2 weeks. Participants relied on us for direction, encouragement and support in both participation and socialization. Some structure was necessary during this time including; maintaining the same time and day each week, and developing ground rules in Week 1 that were later referred to as needed, particularly in times of conflict.

2 Innovative Resources, Bendigo, Australia.

Participants developed a schedule for each week including the time of the coffee break. All groups decided to open each workshop with the education/ discussion time followed by the brainstorming that was used to begin the song writing process. Brainstorming activities began in Week 2. In Week 1 all groups looked at Maslow's Hierarchy of Needs (Maslow 1971) and discussion centred around the needs of parents and their children. For many participants this was the first time that this topic had been discussed.

In Week 2 the group discussed and brainstormed the effects of their child abuse whilst in Week 3 the discussion focused around the effect of their child abuse on their parenting. These weeks formed the beginning of the song writing process. By Week 4, the three groups were beginning to identify themes for further exploration in their group song writing.

Middle stages of the group

During the middle stages, song writing predominated with group members eager and able to recognize that they can create their group songs. The majority of members wrote verses or added to their journal during the week. Most had never written before, and certainly had never written about their feelings, either about their abuse in their childhood and/or adulthood or about parenting of their children. In this stage music listening became less important to group members. Participants wanted to focus on the task of writing their song. For some group members this was an individual song, while others were contributing to group songs. Tears, anger and laughter were all part of the group process. Hope for their children was the driving force during this stage.

Initially most group members felt daunted at the prospect of writing a group song but by the middle stages many were beginning to write a verse and some were requesting to write their own song. At this stage, recording was not discussed or used. In the middle stage, group members were the motivators and task setters. As facilitators, our role became more of guidance, validation and support.

In the beginning of the writing process participants could not decide what they could write about. Over the development of the group, themes were developed, sentences were put together and excitement grew as songs were slowly emerging. Around Weeks 8–10, in all three groups, there was a period of frustration where the activity or creative flow became 'stuck'.

There was always one week where nothing was achieved with regards to the song creations. All involved, including the facilitators were left feeling drained and frustrated at not being able to move forward. In two of the groups we would sit and debate over the inclusion of one word for anything up to 45 min.

For Group 2, the word in question was 'that'. All words became important for the group members as these words were reflecting their lives and feelings. Over the time, we realized this was a pattern in the process of the development of their songs. Usually by the following week there was always a breakthrough and that simply could be restructuring a sentence, use of another word or redefining the theme of the song. The flow again resurged and the group became re-energized and more strongly committed.

As members grew in confidence and trust their individuality began to emerge. Task orientated members became frustrated with others who enjoyed the socialization, while for many of the group members who were experiencing isolation this social contact was crucially important. Conflict therefore emerged in this storming phase of group work (Tuckman 1965). It was important that conflict remained open until resolved and not ignored or minimized. Some members displayed their wish to dominate adding to the conflict in this storming stage. It was exciting to watch the group members become empowered and to begin to find their voice but at the same time, it added a new dimension to the group dynamics and particular support was needed from the facilitators to reduce the possibility of fragmentation of the group.

Terminating stages of the group

The terminating phase of the parenting programme occurred over the final three sessions. Parenting became the focus of the group discussions with an increased self-awareness bringing the focus of discussions back to the participant's children. It was a sad as well as an exciting period; sad because the groups were going to finish but at the same time exciting as all the work and time was beginning to pay off as the songs were being finalized.

Rehearsal and recording were also part of the process in this final stage. Rehearsal time was usually difficult. Tension over the presentation of the songs and verse arose. It was a time of friction and at times that friction was focused on the facilitators, particularly the music therapist.

Some members were anxious about singing whilst others wanted more input into the way the song was to be performed on the CD. Again, it was a time where much support was needed to ensure all participants were having their say not only those who were more dominant. Unlike the later stage of the group process where all were working together, during the rehearsal process it felt at times that members were perhaps obstructing the progress and being deliberately resistant. We often questioned whether this was some kind of personal sabotage as they mostly felt unworthy of this achievement or fear of exposing their deepest and most personal self to an unknown audience. The predominant message group members had received growing up was that they were no good, and that is what they had come to believe about themselves. Whatever the reason it was again a time of frustration and bewilderment for everyone.

Reflections on the tangible product of a CD of songs

At every stage of the group process, the women were given choices as to how they wished to record the songs, and if they still wanted to record. It was never a priority to get to the recording stage but it was an opportunity that seemed to motivate group members. However, it was a daunting process for many of the participants. Huge headphones, microphones, a male stranger sitting at the controls in this darkened studio brought reality to the wishes expressed. This stage of the group was probably the one which differed the most between the three groups of parents, with decisions about who would sing with who, what kind of support was needed individually during recording, and emotions running high, all playing their part. Each group went through this process in a different way, and we, as facilitators, needed to be extremely flexible and available during this time. Overall though, each participant decided to attend the recording sessions and contribute to the recording of the CD in whatever way they felt comfortable.

The importance of the recording stage of the group process was always felt by facilitators and confirmed by participants during subsequent research interviews and focus groups. Participants reported the importance of leaving the group with the CD as something tangible to keep. It gave them a sense of achievement and the feeling that all those weeks had not been wasted. Because they created it, the CD became their means to reflect and deal with their past, and it became a symbol for their pain, memories, struggles and their survival.

Participants reflected the opportunities that creating the CD had provided for them and what it meant in the following statements provided at evaluation:

I am able to take something home. Something good has come out of something bad.

You don't just walk away at the end of it with nothing but memories. We actually have something tangible that we can keep forever.

When I need to deal with it I am also able to listen to the CD and reflect on this group. I finally have something tangible to take home.

You know it is something that you have made, there forever. You recognise the words, hey that's my bit. You can play those songs that mean the most to you.

[It is] a feeling of achievement, like we have made something. It is like pay day.

Project outcomes

We subsequently completed research studies on this project (Bruderer 2007; Day 2007). Both studies aimed to understand the experiences of the women about this unique type of parenting programme. Helen's research focused on collecting data relating to the experiences of participants at the time of the project through focus groups and questionnaires. Toni's study was retrospective and involved interviewing five of the participants approximately 3 years after the project was completed.[3] Many positive outcomes were reported for the women participants and their children at the time of the programme, so it was important to us to find out more about how it was experienced by them, and discover, whether in fact, they felt the experience had been worthwhile in the longer term and, most importantly, had led them to feel more confident as parents. We wanted to continue to allow the voices of the women who participated in this project to be heard, as they had been in the project, and we felt that researching the project from their perspective, was a way to assure this. Therefore the voices of the women are reported throughout.

Participants reported positive outcomes from participating in the parenting programme that used music. They reported that the group was a safe, sharing and supportive environment, stating that they had a social, encouraging and productive experience. Participants described the use of song writing as a vehicle for self-expression and a means for connecting participants together. The women reported the significance of getting their message out to society, educating society about abuse through the creation of their songs. Participants reported the importance of developing a tangible product (the CD), stating they came with nothing but were leaving with something.

The parenting programme participants reported gaining increased skills, awareness, confidence and coping skills both in their parenting and personally. They also indicated positive changes in family communication. With a better understanding of their self and reduced anger as a result of their participation, participants stated they were better able to break the cycle of violence. Some of the comments from women involved that demonstrate their experiences included:

It makes you aware of the cycle repeating. Over the past eleven weeks I have become a lot more confident. I am the one who has the power most of the time.

It helps me to understand myself and therefore helps me in my parenting. I have become more assertive. I am a better parent and now I can speak up for my kids.

---

[3] The project was approved by The University of Queensland Behavioural and Social Science Ethical Review Committee and consent to interview participants was obtained prior to conducting the interviews.

I am not as angry as I was when I first started. I have dealt with a lot of emotions and issues. That is why it has helped me. I noticed I was a very angry person.

I am more aware of what my consequences can lead to. I can stop myself when I get really angry.

It has been hard and I've needed help and I asked for help so that I wouldn't hurt my child.

It's been strange to come to a group that doesn't agree with violence when everyone I know does. It puts everything back into perspective and sees that violence is wrong.

Women in this study reported that the song writing process within the safety of a group played an important therapeutic role for them as survivors of childhood abuse. Song writing, and the subsequent performance of their work, developed their awareness of the impact of childhood abuse on their lives. The process allowed for self-expression and emotional release and increased their self-esteem through providing a sense of achievement. Vicky commented:

I was really amazed how it really helped to bring out feelings, bring back memories and how to express myself. I really didn't think it would help at all but it really helped. I was really surprised . . . It just felt like you were a part of something more than yourself and it stops being so personal and intimate and it was for a good reason and it was just easier to say things.

She continued:

I took it all out on my son all the time and when it finally sunk in, sort of like an epiphany or something, I thought I can't do this to him anymore, it's not his fault. I realized I'm doing exactly the same thing that was done to me . . . I'm treating him like that too . . . It helped me realise that it can't keep going that way. Other people were talking about it . . . yeh. It [the abuse] *was going to keep going forever.*

Song writing provided a forum for therapeutic work that was at times emotionally painful and challenging, but it also allowed participants to feel that their voices had been heard. The women in this project reported that by telling their stories through song, people listened more than if they had used spoken words only. This is of paramount importance for adult survivors of childhood abuse as they were often not believed or 'heard' as children (Herman 1997; Austin 2001).

Maria commented:

It's one thing for people to hear you talk about your experience, but music is powerful. Yeh, and it just seems more. It's got more feeling than just telling people–I've been in domestic violence, I've been abused as a child. People listen more.

Maria's reflections on the recording process indicated that she found the process emotional, but at the same time she also experienced a sense of power:

> . . . there were a lot of different feelings . . . It was also moving . . . I was very excited that I was going to be recording my song that I wrote . . . I wanted to sing it myself even though I've got a terrible voice!

Most participants experienced the song writing process as providing a sense of pride and achievement. Importantly then, these participants revealed that by achieving success in the song writing and performing processes, they experienced an increased self-esteem. Kelly stated:

> We'd actually done it mate . . . us bunch of girls had the feelings about ourselves that we couldn't really see anything through and we'd actually done it and we'd done a bloody good job of it too. We were pretty impressed, pretty proud of ourselves. I've definitely shared it around, been very proud of it most definitely.

Further more, during the follow-up research interviews, all participants reported to have listened to their songs since the completion of the programme. Not all participants continued to listen regularly but they suggested a variety of reasons for listening to their songs in the present day. They have shared their songs with friends, partners and children to help them understand their childhood experiences and how these experiences have affected who they are as people now; and because they are proud of their achievements. Their reports also indicate that songs have been shared as a way of strengthening relationships with significant others, thus indicating that they continue to have therapeutic potential.

Kelly stated:

> We'd grown up in families that you know everything was kept behind closed doors and silenced and you don't go telling people about that sort of stuff and it's got to be brought out for the fact of it educates people . . . this is real life stuff, this is what really happens that nobody ever hears about . . . everyone can open their lives a little bit and not be so judgmental of other people.

Tracy commented:

> It was good to share it with other people . . . it helps them to understand a bit more . . . I've been thinking about airing it on local radio.

Vicky reflected on the way sharing the songs on the CD contributed to strengthening significant relationships:

> Togetherness with people . . . It feels like you actually trust them a bit more because it shows that you trust them to let them into you.

Future directions

Many lessons were learned during this project. Participants advocated for longer running groups or increased hours each session. Future programmes could possibly be enhanced with body work such as movement, and training in voice and/or singing.

Attachment with their children was a key concern for many participants, and this was of concern to the facilitators also. Most participants acknowledged they had no experience of play in their childhood. Future programmes are recommended to consider providing time for the mothers only as well as for parents and children together.

Further programmes would need to continue to be responsive to the needs of the participants, and have a flexible approach to the structure of the sessions. Additionally there are other target groups that could benefit from this type of programme such as fathers who have similar childhoods, indigenous parents and young parents. Longitudinal studies of the parents would enhance the knowledge of the benefits of such programmes and assist in future development of programmes.

Roles of facilitators: combining music therapy and social work

It was difficult to define the roles of the social worker and music therapist apart from the music therapist holding musical expertise required to assist the participants to create the music for their songs. The groups were genuinely co-facilitated in that both of us supported and encouraged the members in the creation of the lyrics to their songs. There was a common purpose, and we shared similar values, communication styles and senses of humour. One of the more challenging areas was finding a shared professional language by which to communicate. Many times we were discussing the same point or had the same opinion but did not realize it due to the terminology we were using.

Technically the social worker's role involved supporting and educating about issues relating to parenting and the music therapist's role revolved around song writing and recording. However, in practicality the process was so intertwined that no clear role emerged. It was more important to support each other and work as a team.

Understanding the dynamics of the groups, and attending sensitively to aspects of the stages and process became an integral part of our learning. Commonalities exist between a vast array of human services disciplines and this was evident with social work and music therapy. To be truly responsive to the needs of participants, looking beyond disciplinary boundaries was required.

The inter-professional experience gained working in this project was both challenging and rewarding. The increased knowledge, experience and skills gained from combining the practice of social work with music therapy were appreciated. This approach not only attracted the attention of a reluctant group of parents, but the collaboration also gave a unique and creative approach to parenting education that offered a range of important benefits to a vulnerable group of parents and their children.

Conclusion

We would like to conclude by acknowledging the strength and courage of all the mothers involved in this project. Their songs give voice to their pain and demonstrate the commitment they hold to have different lives for themselves and their children. As with the first words of this chapter, the final words of this chapter also belong to them.

STOP

Hitting, yelling, swearing, touching, rape, hair pulling, punching and neglect
We are the adult survivors of all those abuses
And whilst they are different, united, we share the one face,
Help us stop the abuse
We all have rights to be educated and loved
We all have rights to feel safe
We all have rights to live without abuse
We all have rights but as kids we didn't know
It's hard to say – STOP!
Smiling happy children that's what you think you see
We children tend to put on masks just for you to see
You'd never listen anyway so why should we try
You'd say it never happened you'd say that I have lied
I know how you feel, I felt it too,
I'll do my best just for you
So you don't have to experience what I did
So you can live your life free from FEAR
How can you love when you've never known love
And hear a child's cry when no-one listened to you
How do you feel another's pain, when it's deep inside of you
I want to heal my life and feel normal for a while
The abuse I suffered as a child has made my life a trial
Help me find a better way to love my child
To change our lives and get through each day
Living with years of abuse has left me feeling empty, incomplete and not whole
So much of my life is a struggle like everything is against me, even my children at times
I do not want to be a mother who nags, screams negates or beats
Instead I turn to my addictions to distance myself from the pain

Providing a sense of relief
I learnt trust was no friend of mine, hope was my only friend I felt each day
My love I hope will be stronger than the rage that swells inside of me
I hope to change and learn new ways from how I have been raised
To be a gentle loving mum to my son, who I see now already mirrors me
We all have rights to be educated and loved
We all have rights to feel safe
We all have rights to live without abuse
We all have rights but as kids we didn't know
It's hard to say – STOP!

© Strength to Strength, 2001

References

Abad, V., and Edwards, J. (2004). Strengthening families: a role for music therapy in contributing to family centred care. *The Australian Journal of Music Therapy*, 15, 3–17.

Amir, D. (1999). Tales from the therapy room. In J. Hibben (ed.) *Inside Music Therapy: Client Experiences.* (Gilsum, NH: Barcelona Publishers)

Amir, D. (2004). Giving trauma a voice: the role of improvisational music therapy in exposing, dealing with and healing a traumatic experience of sexual abuse. *Music Therapy Perspectives*, 22, 96–104.

Anderson, J. (1997). *Social Work with Groups: A Process Model.* (New York: Longman)

Austin, D. (2001). In search of the self: the use of vocal holding techniques with adults traumatised as children. *Music Therapy Perspectives*, 19, 22–30.

Austin, D. (2006). Songs of the self: vocal psychotherapy for adults traumatized as children. In L. Corey (ed.) *Expressive and Creative Arts Methods for Trauma Survivors*, pp. 133–151. (London: Jessica Kingsley)

Australian Association of Social Workers (2002). *Code of Ethics 1999*, 2nd Edn. (Canberra: ACT, Australian Association of Social Workers)

Australian Institute of Health and Welfare (2006). *Child Protection Australia.* Cat. No. CWS 26. (Canberra: Australian Institute of Health and Welfare)

Baker, F., and Wigram, T. (eds) (2005). *Song Writing: Methods, Techniques and Clinical Applications for Music Therapy Clinicians, Educators and Students.* (London: Jessica Kingsley)

Bowes, J. (2000). *Parent's response to parent education and support programs.* National Child Protection Clearinghouse, Newsletter 8 (2). (Melbourne: Australian Institute of Family Studies)

Blundo, R. (2001). Learning strengths-based practice: challenging our personal and professional frames. *Families in Society: The Journal of Contemporary Human Services*, 82, 296–304.

Bruderer, H. (2007). Parenting, Songwriting and Violence: Perceptions of Participants in Three Parenting Groups. Unpublished Masters Thesis, The University of Queensland.

Cassity, M.D., and Theobold, K.A. (1990). Domestic violence: assessment and treatments employed by music therapists. *Journal of Music Therapy*, 27, 179–194.

Chenoweth, L., and McAuliffe, D. (2005). *The Road to Social Work and Human Service Practice: An Introductory Text.* (Victoria: Thomson Learning)

Clendenon-Wallen, J. (1991). The use of music therapy to influence the self-confidence and self-esteem of adolescents who are sexually abused. *Music Therapy Perspectives*, 9, 73–81.

Courtois, C. (2000). Foreword. In S. Gold (ed.) *Not Trauma Alone: Therapy for Child Abuse Survivors in Family and Social Context*. (Philadelphia, PA: Brunner-Routledge)

Dale, P., Davies, M., Morrison, T., and Waters, J. (1989). *Dangerous Families–Assessment and Treatment of Child Abuse*. (London: Tavistock)

Day, T. (2005). Giving a voice to childhood trauma through therapeutic song writing. In F. Baker, and T. Wigram. (eds) *Song Writing: Methods, Techniques and Clinical Applications for Music Therapy Clinicians, Educators and Students*, pp. 82–96. (London: Jessica Kingsley)

Day, T. (2007). A Retrospective Exploration of the Role of Song Writing for Five Women who have Experienced Childhood Abuse. Unpublished Masters Thesis, The University of Queensland.

DiLillo, D., Tremblay, G., and Peterson, L. (2000). Linking childhood sexual abuse and abusive parenting: the mediating role of maternal anger. *Child Abuse and Neglect*, 24, 767–779.

Edgerton, C.D. (1990). Creative group song writing. *Music Therapy Perspectives*, 8, 15–19.

Ethier, L.S., Lacharite, C., and Couture, G. (1995). Childhood adversity, parental stress, and depression of negligent mothers. *Child Abuse and Neglect*, 19, 619–632.

Fergusson, D., Boden, J., and Horwood, J. (2008). Exposure to childhood sexual and physical abuse and adjustment in early adulthood. *Child Abuse and Neglect*, 32, 607–619.

Glassman, U., and Kates, L. (1990). *Group Work: a Humanistic Approach*. (California: Newbury Park)

Haapasalo, J., and Aaltonen, T. (1999). Child abuse potential: how persistent? *Journal of Interpersonal Violence*, 14, 571–585.

Hadley, S. (Ed.) (2006). *Feminist Perspectives in Music Therapy*. (Gilsum, NH: Barcelona)

Hall, K. (2008). Childhood sexual abuse and adult sexual problems: a new view of assessment and treatment. *Feminism and Psychology*, 18, 546–556.

Herman, J. (1997). *Trauma and Recovery*, 2nd Edn. (New York: Basic Books)

Lyons, S. (2000). Make, make, make some music: social group work with mothers and babies together. *Social Work with Groups*, 23, 37–54.

MacIntosh, H.B. (2003). Sounds of healing: music in group work with survivors of sexual abuse. *The Arts in Psychotherapy*, 30, 17–23.

Maltz, W., and Holman, B. (1987). *Incest and Sexuality*. (New York: Lexington)

Maslow, A.H. (1971). *The Farther Reaches of Human Nature*. (Middlesex: Penguin)

Montello, L. (1999). A psychoanalytic music therapy approach to treating adults traumatized as children. *Music Therapy Perspectives*, 17, 74–81.

Mullen, P.E., Martin, J.L., Anderson, J.C., Romons, S.E., and Herbison, G.P. (1996). The long-term impact of the physical, emotional and sexual abuse of children: a community study. *Child Abuse and Neglect*, 20, 7–21.

Nicholson, J.M., Berthelsen, D., Abad, V., Williams, K., and Bradley, J. (2008). Impact of music therapy to promote positive parenting and child development. *Journal of Health Psychology*, 13, 226–238.

NSW Commission for Children and Young People and Bruce Callaghan and Associates. (2000). *New South Wales Interagency Guidelines for Child Protection Intervention*. (Sydney: NSW Government)

O'Brien, W. (1991). Making parent education relevant to vulnerable parents. *Children Australia*, 16, 19–26.

Oldfield, A., and Bunce, L. (2001). 'Mummy can play too . . .': short-term music therapy with mothers and young children. *British Journal of Music Therapy*, 15, 27–35.

Payne, M. (1994). *Modern Social Work Theory: a Critical Introduction.* (London: MacMillan)

Pinquart, M. and Teubert, D. (2010). Effects of parenting education with expectant and new parents: a meta-analysis. *Journal of Family Psychology*, 24, 316–327.

Poole, L., and Tomison, A. (2000). *Preventing child abuse in Australia: some preliminary findings from a National Audit of prevention programs.* Paper presented at the 7th Australian Family Research Conference, Sydney.

Priebe, G. And Svedin, C.(2008). Child sexual abuse is largely hidden from the adult society: an epidemiological study of adolescents' disclosures. *Child Abuse and Neglect*, 32, 1095–1108.

Rogers, P. (1995). Childhood sexual abuse: dilemmas in therapeutic practice. *Music Therapy Perspectives*, 13, 24–30.

Rogers, P. (2003). Working with Jenny: stories of gender, power and abuse. In S. Hadley (ed.) *Psychodynamic Music Therapy: Case Studies*, pp. 123–140. (Gilsum, NH: Barcelona)

Ruscio, A.M. (2001). Predicting the child-rearing practices of mothers sexually abused in childhood. *Child Abuse and Neglect*, 25, 369–387.

Saleeby, D. (Ed.) (1997). *The Strengths Perspective in Social Work Practice*, 2nd Edn. (New York: Longman)

Schuetze, P., and Das Eiden, R. (2005). The relationship between sexual abuse during childhood and parenting outcomes: modeling direct and indirect pathways. *Child Abuse and Neglect*, 29, 645–659.

Scott, D., and O'Neil, D. (1996). *Beyond Child Rescue–Developing Family-Centred Practice at St Luke's.* (Sydney: Allen and Unwin)

Tuckman, B. (1965). Developmental sequence in small groups. *Psychological Bulletin*, 63, 384–399.

Whipple, J., and Lindsey, R. (1999). Music for the soul: a music therapy program for battered women. *Music Therapy Perspectives*, 17, 61–68.

White, M., and Denborough, D. (1998). *Introducing Narrative Therapy–A Collection of Practice Based Writings.* (Adelaide: Dulwich Centre)

Wigram, T. (2005). Songwriting methods–similarities and differences: developing a working model. In F. Baker and T. Wigram (eds) *Song writing: Methods, Techniques and Clinical Applications for Music Therapy Clinicians, Educators and Students*, pp. 246–264. (London: Jessica Kingsley)

Chapter 11

Translating 'infant-directed singing' into a strategy for the hospitalized family

Helen Shoemark

It is 6.30 in the evening, and a mother stands in her living room, obviously weary from the day's care of her new baby boy. He is now snuggled in the crook of her arm, his face relaxed as he finally ebbs towards sleep. The mother sings the same few lines of lullaby over and over willing him to sleep deeply so she can gently convey him to bed and finally to rest herself.

In the Special Care Nursery, a mother returns her baby to bed, unthreading his lines and tubes from her fingers. The baby boy cannot slip into the sleep he so desperately needs because his breathing is tortured by the spit rising in his trachea. The nurse slides the fine tube into his trachea to suction out the fluid, momentarily preventing the baby from breathing. His mother chants a gentle reassurance as he begins to howl at this physically distressing procedure. When they've finished, the mother silently sighs as he instantly drops into deep sleep. She sits and stares at him knowing that it is only 30 min until his sleep will be disrupted again to repeat the traumatic procedure.

Introduction

The experience of mothering a newborn infant in a hospital is far from the reality of being a parent at home. The mother in hospital is powerless to change the experience of trauma her infant feels each time life-saving suctioning takes place. Worse still, the infant comes to know that she is powerless too.

It might optimistically be assumed that a music therapist helps the family in hospital by encouraging the mother to use singing to help her baby recover. However, the assumption is not so straightforward. How can the 'ordinary' experience of singing serve this extraordinary situation? It may be natural to presume that the phenomenon of infant-directed singing (Trehub et al. 1993a) can be directly translated to support the hospital experience of the mother–infant dyad. However, there are a number of considerations that require attention in the real-world applications of infant-directed singing in a hospital setting.

This chapter provides an exploration of the possibilities for the music therapist employing infant-directed singing both with the infant's family, and also directly with the infant. First the experience of the healthy infant in the context of the infant's family will be presented, and then an exploration of the hospital experience for a newborn infant and family will create a picture about the potential and value of music therapy in this context. Finally, the chapter will focus on how and why infant-directed singing provides a simple yet potent experience for the developing infant.

Infant-directed speech

The foetus is able to hear and recognize sounds to which he has been repeatedly exposed *in utero*, such as family voices, and particularly the mother's voice (De Casper and Fifer 1980; Fifer and Moon 1994; Hepper 1994). This 'transnatal' learning, as Moon and Fifer (2000) have described it, means that the infant is already receptive to sounds such as his or her family's voices and these will be the most familiar and thus potent auditory experiences that the infant can use at and after birth.

Newborn infants show their recognition of voices with a brief deceleration of the heart rate, called an orienting response (Ockleford et al. 1988). Infants less than 24 h old are able to discriminate between a range of voices. Using their orienting response they are able to demonstrate to researchers their strongest preference for the mother's voice followed by the father's voice before a stranger's voice. The importance of this finding is that as the music therapist, I am a stranger to the infant and therefore I must consider that my voice holds far less interest than the voice of the infant's mother.

The most important acoustical feature of familiar voices is the fundamental frequency, or pitch of the voice (Spence and Freeman 1996). Infant-directed speech can be described as the 'sing-song' way of speaking that adults adopt with infants. The key features of infant-directed speech are a raised pitch, an expanded range of pitches, and exaggerated intonation contours (Fernald and Kuhl 1987). It was Fernald who proposed that since infants cannot understand the information content of speech, the communicative intention is embedded in the pulse and intonation aspects of speech called 'prosody'. Fernald called this the 'melody of mothers' speech' (Fernald 1989 p. 1497). This recognition of the musicality of speech directed toward infants has entrenched musical vocabulary into the language to describe mother–infant communication.

Infant-directed speech includes specific melody-like patterns that offer different information to the infant with specific melodic patterns closely aligned to maternal care-giving tasks (Stern et al. 1982; Fernald, 1989). Papoušek and Papoušek found specific vocal patterns had a consistent form for specific functions when talking to infants aged 2 months. Rising contours were associated with encouraging turn-taking and evaluating infant state; falling and bell-shaped contours with rewarding; falling contours with soothing; a 'cuckoo call' type of bell-shaped contour with encouraging visual contact; and level and bell-shaped contours with discouraging unfavourable behaviour (Papoušek and Papoušek 1991). This research has supported the growing appreciation that high-pitched, expanded melodic contours in infant-directed speech elicit and maintain infant attention.

Infant-directed singing

Infant-directed singing is similar to infant-directed speech in that adults alter the way they sing when they are singing to infants and children (Trehub et al. 1993a, 1993b). At an obvious level, different types of songs serve different purposes. Parents sing play songs to encourage their infant's active interest, while lullabies encourage the infant to settle and go to sleep.

When adults listen to recordings of parents singing lullabies they can distinguish when the parent is singing to their infant, or when they are singing a lullaby without their infant present. This difference is even able to be spotted when the lullabies are from different cultures (Trainor et al. 1997). When parents sing to their infant, they sing at a slower tempo, with more energy in the lower frequencies, with longer pauses between the sung lines, and with a higher pitch and more vibrato. Even when mothers, fathers and other children pretend to sing to their infant, listeners are able to tell whether the infant is present or not (Trehub and Schellenberg 1995).

When parents sing to their infants the key feature is a higher emotional engagement (Trehub et al. 1997). This means that both mothers and fathers sing more expressively, using a higher pitch level and slower tempo (Trehub et al. 1997; Trainor et al. 2000). If the song is playful then the singing is more 'brilliant, clipped, and rhythmic', while lullabies are more 'airy, smooth, and soothing' (Rock et al. 1999 p. 527). Mothers particularly emphasize the temporal structure of song, elongating the mid point of the phrase and the end of the phrase to help infants process the song just as they would a spoken phrase in infant-directed speech, thus offering the infant additional rehearsal of key processing skills (Longhi 2009).

This research is the starting point to understand how the music therapist can make use of naturally occurring parent–infant patterns in clinical work with infants, and also in helping mothers to see how they might find a way to use their own voice with their infant. In working with hospitalized infants in music therapy interactions I use these defined features to inform how I sing.

Infant learning: self-regulation and interactive regulation

One function of the human brain is to seek order and patterns, to make sense of the world (Schore 1994). In order to maintain physical survival, this regulation is evident in the infant's control of the earliest states of hunger, sleep, arousal and social contact. The newborn infant quickly learns how to have his or her basic needs met through crying, and within a few weeks moves into other kinds of interaction with his carers beginning the important journey of learning how to be with another person. The infant learns to regulate the amount of stimulation he receives from those around him or her, decipher its value and determine how he or she will respond. The infant is able to integrate information across several sensory modalities essential for normal development (Stern 1985; Crown et al. 2002). Within weeks, the infant begins to develop the intricate capability to regulate all aspects of self which in turn drives the infant to make sense of the stimulation offered, as if the infant was 'biologically prepared to engage in activity to stimulate his own brain' (Beebe et al. 2000).

Infants develop 'micro-regulatory social-emotional process' (Tronick 1998) through opportunities for both feedback and contribution to the partnership with another person (Beebe et al. 2000). The give and take in their interactions is called 'mutual' or 'interactive' regulation (Beebe and Lachmann 1994; Tronick 1998; Beebe et al. 2005). These interactions include the infant's own behaviour (self-regulation) and the infant's partner's behaviour (interactive regulation). The shared responsibility for successful interaction is usually achieved implicitly, but further examination provides evidence of key elements which are useful for the music therapist who is consciously creating a therapeutic intervention.

At the age of 6 weeks, the full-term healthy infant is able to coordinate his or her interaction with an adult partner using visual gaze (Crown et al. 2002). Crown and his research team observed that strangers worked harder than mothers to coordinate interactions with the infant. This confirmed that 'the greater the degree of uncertainty, novelty or challenge, the greater the need to make the interaction predictable' (Beebe et al. 2000). Jaffe et al. (2001) also showed that mid-range coordination was the infant's optimal level for attachment with mothers and strangers, but that high infant–stranger coordination was optimal for cognition.

The impact of being born with a major medical problem that requires surgical or other medical care places this fine-tuned developmental process in jeopardy. Knowledge of these developmental factors is therefore an important part of the music therapist's repertory. The therapist can then use them to consciously construct and respond to the interactive timing of the medically fragile newborn infant.

The experience of hospitalization

The ability of the newborn to achieve balance relies on the successful achievement of three tasks: (1) establishing homeostasis through self-regulation of state; (2) processing, storing and organizing multiple stimuli; and (3) establishing a reciprocal relationship with a primary caretaker and with the environment (Kaminski and Hall 1996). For the medically fragile newborn infant most of his or her energy is used trying to establish and maintain the homeostasis, or stability, of various body systems. The infant may suffer from prolonged periods of discomfort or pain with associated wind, nausea, vomiting, or excessive oral secretions caused by the medical condition. These may cause ongoing or frequent periods in the 'active alert' state when the infant is restless, with agitated movements and grimaces, or in 'crying' state, which can magnify the energy expenditure of an infant by as much as 200%, and may cause an increase in an infant's basal metabolic rate (Rose and Mayer 1968). The infant may also spend periods of time under the effects of medication for pain relief, or under sedation/muscle relaxant to minimize distress while repairing from precarious surgeries.

The medical care of the infant is planned to promote physical healing which involves the supervision of many tasks for which the infant might otherwise be responsible. Seeking food is replaced by scheduled feeding, rarely at the breast or from a bottle, often through a nasogastric tube, sometimes directly into the stomach through a gastrostomy tube and in some cases via a special solution administered intravenously. The consequence of this is that the infant loses his or her opportunity to both determine his or her own needs and to explore how to successfully demand to have them met. Also, despite system improvements to provide a consistency in care teams, the reality is that care and interaction is offered by an array of people with varying patterns of sensitivity to the infant's non-medical needs. Programmes such as the Newborn Individualized Developmental Care and Assessment Program (NIDCAP) place the infant's needs at the centre of the care protocol, building a process that intends to be more consistently responsive to the infant (Als 1996). Such a programme requires a major shift in the philosophy which permeates an entire unit of care professionals, and as such can be slow to implement consistently.

The work undertaken in this music therapy programme is based on the transactional model of child development which suggests that no one factor is responsible for a child's development, but rather it is the result of the interplay between a variety of factors (Sameroff and Fiese 2000). When enough risk factors accumulate, the child is at greater risk of a poor developmental outcome (Sameroff et al. 1998). The infant's healthy development will be best supported when parents are able to provide ongoing experiences of mutual regulation within a stable and nurturing environment (Lillas and Turnbull 2009). Using these ideas, the purpose of interpersonal interventions for the hospitalized newborn infant is to sustain the family's ability to provide that stable and nurturing context amidst the barrage of complex medical care.

Experiences of the hospitalized family

Parents have reported that being in the neonatal intensive care unit (NICU) with their infant is like being in an 'alien world' or being spectators in their own lives, oscillating between hope and hopelessness (Hall 2005). The greatest stress is reported to be a change in their role as parents, with a lack of choice and control, and feelings of intimidation, grief and inadequacy (Seidemen et al. 1997; McGrath 2001). Many hospitals now ensure parents are offered the opportunity to bathe, feed, dress and attend to any other elements of care that they might have done at home with their baby. When these are possible, they can preserve close physical contact and interaction which are both significant experiences in building parent–infant attachment (Carol Newnham, infant neuropsychologist, personal communication 2006). However, medical care and monitoring regimes, periods of sedation, and extended periods of sleep may prevent several of these tasks. Additionally, infants may not be receptive to parental attention or may offer behavioural cues which are difficult to interpret. This may lead to the parent being unsure of how to proceed. The pleasure that could be shared may be seriously disrupted, causing a disturbance to the development of greater intimacy in the first few months of life. Clinicians have suggested that services which offer containment to parents' emotional reactions and anxieties can help parents in turn to contain and support their infant (Parker et al. 1992; Miles et al. 1999; Hurst 2001; Harris 2005).

In a study of music therapy with vulnerable infants, Malloch and his research team examined what occurred when a music therapist consciously employed the attributes of mother–infant speech and singing with medically fragile newborn infants three times per week for up to 4 weeks (Malloch et al. in press). The result was a significant effect on the infant's neuropsychological development particularly noted by a reduction in irritability and crying, causing scores on the Neurobehavioral Assessment of the Preterm Infant (NAPI) to improve, while the scores for the infants in the control group actually deteriorated. That the music therapist's singing was so clinically effective was perhaps not surprising in light of previous research findings that strangers' efforts to regulate their communication with 6-week-old infants resulted in better coordinated timing (Crown et al. 2002), and that in the case of singing to older infants (6–9 months), the infants had higher cognitive scores when the music therapist sang to them rather than their own mother (de l'Etoile 2006). What was surprising was that the NAPI scores for the infants in the control group actually deteriorated, suggesting that the experience of being hospitalized had negatively impacted on the infants' neuropsychological development.

The psychosocial status of the infant in the context of the family warrants attention. O'Gorman (2007) has referred to attachment theory (Bowlby 1969; Ainsworth et al. 1978) to identify the importance of the music therapist being able to support a mother's sensitivity to her infant's cues and the amount and quality of interaction with her infant. My duty as a music therapist is therefore to find approachable supportive strategies that the family can use to interact with their baby. Given that (a) infant-directed singing is a preferred stimulus for the newborn infant, which is supportive and responsive to observed facial, gestural and vocal cues, and (b) even as a stranger, the music therapist can consciously and delicately manipulate the known elements of successful interaction to 'be' with the infant, there is potential for the infant to safely accept music therapy and positively impact upon the infant's neuropsychological well-being.

In lieu of contrary evidence it is reasonable to assume that the medically fragile infant's fundamental musicality is intact. This pathway to human contact is a powerful avenue by which the infant can still access and respond to the world. Despite painful experiences, invasive treatment and uncomfortable monitoring, many infants can usually still hear and use early gestures and sounds of emotional expression. Singing is uniquely positive in its expression.

When provided as a contingently responsive stimulation, it is an experience that acknowledges the infant's behavioural cues, and enhances the infant's interpersonal capability without taxing his or her regulatory system. With these accumulated factors, the potential is even greater:

> The neonate's experience of music is not ultimately that of being impacted upon, or influenced by, a set of discreet sound stimuli – it is the experience of wholeness, or health, through sounds shared in a uniquely human way, through human contact. (Abrams *et al.* 2000 p. 38)

It is proposed then that music therapy offers a way for parents, or the therapist, to provide contingent singing to create a unique avenue for infant well-being and development.

Music therapy in an Australian Neonatal Unit

Since 1996 I have provided clinical service to the Neonatal Unit (NNU) at The Royal Children's Hospital Melbourne (RCH). This unit is a 24-bed, level 4 (highest level) NNU with approximately 550 admissions per year. Patients are referred from level 3 perinatal centres both in Melbourne and interstate; maternity hospitals throughout Victoria, neighbouring states and the hospital's Emergency Department (The Royal Children's Hospital Melbourne 2010). The infants referred to this service have a range of complex medical and surgical problems. The unit is based on a family-centred care approach (Griffin 2006) which considers the infant's family to be the primary unit of care, including parents in all aspects of decision making and care of their infant. Infants are often admitted for anything from a few days for tests or simple procedures through to many weeks or months, requiring an effective range of services to accommodate the infant's extraordinary start to life. Music therapy is integrated into the services of two care teams; the psychosocial, and the developmental therapy. The psychosocial team includes social workers, infant mental health specialists, care managers, medical consultant, representatives from the developmental therapy team, and the music therapist. In this team music therapy is used to support parents through partnership to understand their infant and their own potency to parent a sick newborn infant. The developmental therapy team includes a music therapist, physiotherapists, speech therapists, and occupational therapists. Music therapy is employed to support the infant directly with recorded music to support transition from wake to sleep, and developmental opportunities for self and mutual regulation (Shoemark 2006). Across both teams, the infant remains in the context of the family.

We are beginning to understand that fathers experience the hospitalization of a newborn baby differently from the mothers (Fegran et al. 2008). In the context of an Australian NICU, caring for infants in hospital largely remains the role of the mother. The mother is still physically recovering from the birth but is most likely to still be available during the day to attend to her infant, while the father often needs to return to work, maintaining financial security for the family and possibly saving any available leave time for when his baby returns home. Because of this, mothers are most commonly stated in the text below as the person with whom I partner in this work although I do also work with fathers, holding them in mind when they are absent and encouraging their participation when they are present.

Music therapy with families

The common picture of neonatal music therapy is that the music therapist sings to the baby without the parent present, or with a parent looking on or receiving some instruction from the music therapist. This scenario locates the therapist in the role as 'expert', and the infant as 'the patient' or client. In family-centred practice, the parent and infant are considered to hold the primary relationship, while the therapist holds a supportive external role. As Winnicott noted 'there is no such thing as a baby' (1964 p. 88), but rather there is always an infant with a mother, a father and an extended family. The client is not the infant nor the mother (or other carer), but always the mother–infant dyad or indeed the infant and family in triad with the therapist. Even in situations when music therapy may occur without the parents, the music therapist must hold in mind that the infant is part of the family group. So the infant's ability to 'be' with the therapist is mediated through the infant's location in his or her family.

Working primarily with the infant's parent

Assumptions held by practitioners about parents' ability to consciously access an intuitive process such as singing are problematic when parents are enduring extraordinary events. Blumenfeld and Eisenfeld (2006) found that fewer than 20% of mothers who had initially agreed to participate in their study in a NICU actually completed the described protocol of singing to their premature babies while breastfeeding. Mothers noted scheduling difficulties and excessive anxiety about their infant as factors in choosing not to sing, but also reported shyness and inhibition about singing in the NICU environment. This suggests that a therapeutic intervention to support mothers to translate singing into this environment is needed in order to achieve the benefits that singing can offer.

Amidst the initial crisis and long-term stress of hospitalization most parents do not have additional energy to bring their own musicality or musical background to the fore.[1] The task of the music therapist then is to present ways in which music addresses any current stated concerns or some of the issues that families are known to face in the hospital.

In our first meeting, I will talk to the mother about her use of music throughout her pregnancy, giving both an opportunity for me to understand her music use and preferences and to potentially offer the mother affirmation about her own successful employment of recorded music for relaxation. This is a safe starting point which provides entry into the prospect of sharing music with the newborn baby. Once a basis for using music is established, I can begin to facilitate a parent's engagement with her or his own musical capabilities and an awareness that her or his infant's musicality offers clear cues about what is liked and disliked. The music therapist may also call on the parent's own childhood experience of music which was hopefully a positive experience of safety, but if not, then music therapy may not be a useful strategy for the dyad in this time frame. Reference to simple, commonly known songs can often elicit a repertoire of songs long forgotten for the first time parent. Reflection on songs shared with other children can raise memories, particularly for the mother, of her ability to nurture her babies.

The suggestion that the mother might sing to her infant in hospital is most commonly met with the mother's trepidation and self-effacing comments such as 'Oh the baby will really be in trouble if I sing' or 'Everyone will leave if I sing'. It has been rare for me to find a mother who welcomes the opportunity to sing. However this attitude is quickly mediated with key information which verifies the pivotal role of the mother's voice. The research which outlines the baby's ability to recognize his own mother's voice from another woman's voice (DeCasper and Fifer 1980), is the information which mothers find most powerful. The notion that no one else's voice is as meaningful to her baby as hers is, holds great authority and may stand in counterbalance to the mother's perceived loss of status as the nurturing caregiver of her child. The research to indicate that speaking arouses an infant's attention and singing holds it (Nakata and Trehub 2004) fascinates parents in the possibility that there are two distinctively meaningful activities for which they can use their voice. The notion that humming is as meaningful as singing as it retains the melodic content, is a relief to those parents who are overwhelmed by the idea of singing in the seemingly public space of the hospital room.

The fantasy of the perfect newborn infant commonly includes an expectation of music for the baby (Shoemark and Dearn 2008). The potential of a triadic relationship with parent and infant is an expanded capacity to rebuild moments

---

[1] There are always exceptions to this in the parent who is her/himself inherently musical or even a musician.

of joyful experience through the attuned interplay. I serve as a facilitator, container and witness to the contingent interaction of the dyad, affirming the reality of what transpires and confirming or enhancing the mother's judgement of the situation. This serves as a source of empathy and satisfaction for both partners. Sometimes there are serious mismatches between mother and infant. For example, the mother notes with dismay or disgust that her baby will not look at her. I can return to the knowledge base to explain to the mother why such events occur. In the case that the infant looks away when she starts to sing, I can reframe the response as a positive strategy to regulate the amount of stimulation the infant receives. With this explanation the parent has another explanation rather than the rejection she had imagined, thus reducing or deflecting possible negative influence to the parent's sense of self in the unfolding dyadic interplay.

Perhaps most significantly, I can acknowledge the infant as a whole child who does not need to be 'fixed' or made 'better' (Shoemark and Dearn 2008). In the following story, the only music I provided was to support a new mother and her own mother in their attempt to recall the lyrics of a song they had shared long ago. My more significant contribution was instead to merge my knowledge of mother–infant singing to the apparent needs and style of the mother.

Hilary, Lucy, and Nancy: intergenerational song memory

Hilary's mother Lucy was very pleased to meet me and discuss how to apply music to their situation. Lucy was an accountant, and as I spoke, she took meticulous notes. She spoke lightly of such note-taking as being an occupational hazard, and I affirmed that it was a great idea when there were so many things to remember. When I suggested singing, Lucy stopped and looked at me to ask 'But what would I sing? I don't know any songs.' I looked to Lucy's mother, Nancy, who had been standing quietly on the other side of Hilary's bed and suggested that this is where grandmothers were a wonderful resource. Hilary's grandma thought for a moment and offered 'Hey-di-ho' as a song they'd enjoyed together. 'Oh yes, that's right how does it go?' asked Lucy. Grandma began to sing and as she faltered with the lyrics, I joined in to help. Lucy laughed as she frantically began to write down the lyrics, 'How will I remember these?' she said. Later that day, I left a laminated 'cheat sheet' of lyrics by Hilary's bed for the six songs we had discussed. After the weekend when I arrived on the ward, Lucy and Hilary were waiting out in the hallway for the medical rounds to be finished in their shared room. Lucy was smiling and called down the corridor to me, 'Frere Jacques is our absolute favourite, she will listen to it for ages!' As I got closer she said 'Three green and speckled frogs has become two dirty and smelly nappies . . .'. Lucy had not only found her repertoire, she had found playful joy with her precious daughter.

The significant functional step here as therapist was to hold back from singing, allowing Lucy to be the one who brought music into Hilary's life. Lucy was attentive and attuned to Hilary, but apprehensive about what to do with her. She only needed appropriate knowledge and devices for recall of repertoire to open up the possibility of singing to her daughter. Additionally, Lucy and her mother reconnected to their own relationship as mother and child, with Nancy offering her resources at a challenging time.

Initiating something new and unfamiliar might not be possible for the parent on her or his own, but in the expanded capability of the therapeutic triad (Tronick 1998) simple moments can provide a powerful turning point to facilitate parent and infant engagement. Episodes of shared singing and modelling may serve a purpose if sensitively structured.

Working directly with the infant

For an array of reasons, parents may not be present during the infant's wakeful periods. Through negotiated partnership with the parents, the music therapist may offer the infant direct interaction which respects the primary relationship of the family. Where the parents are emotionally and physically available partners to their infants but unable to be at the hospital during wakeful periods, it is important to acknowledge to the parents that the music therapist does not serve in their place or as a surrogate, but as an additional source for attuned interplay. Where parents are emotionally or physically unavailable to their infants, such as the case where the mother feels unable to bond with her baby in case the baby dies, or culturally based hesitation where the sick baby is seen as a punishment from God, the music therapist can provide an intersubjective experience which offers companionship (Trevarthen 2001). However caution is needed that the therapist does not experience themselves as 'saving' the baby from the inadequate family situation. It is vital to understand that the therapeutic relationship is a transient one, offered only to 'hold' the potential of attachment for the infant until the infant's family is available.

In singing directly to medically fragile newborns, the key difference from naturally occurring interaction is the music therapist's intentions in the interplay. The therapeutic focus is on producing change only for the infant such as in their state, and awareness capability for example, and while change might occur in the therapist, it is not the goal of the work. The therapist brings their full knowledge, including personal and professional insight to interpret the process and make decisions about how to proceed. It is essential that the therapist acknowledges their own journey in coming to this work (Stewart 2001) and understands those experiences which inform their skills, sensibilities and interpretations. Supervision is therefore strongly recommended to support the process of reflecting on the work.

In sessions with very young infants or otherwise socially unavailable infants, the focus of the music therapy interaction is sensory support. This is particularly important for an infant whose usual pattern of mostly sleeping may be disturbed by pain or procedures. I consciously employ elements of infant-directed singing and therefore to differentiate it from naturally occurring or spontaneous process, I have called this method 'contingent singing' (Shoemark and Dearn 2008). This might involve a vocal or speech pattern which appeals to the infant such as a repeated sound like 'ch, ch' or 'oh, oh, oh' which is quite bright and clipped in attack and timbre, regular in its rhythm and with an extremely limited range of pitches (Shoemark 2008). The intention is to introduce a stimulus which will cause the infant to attend to me. This will be evident in their behaviour such as becoming still to listen, or changing from sleep to alert. Once attention is established, I use the same intonated line, tempo, timbre, and attack, modulating this as the infant demonstrates more or less interest. This chanting also offers the music therapist or a parent a generous range of subtle variation to protect and support the infant.

The experience of the socially available infant is still mediated by physical restriction of positioning, for example infants with a cardiac condition may be placed on one side only to improve function. Limited scope of action may also reduce availability, for example infants with a replogle tube to drain secretion from their oesophagus, can only be raised to about a 45° angle. Other factors may be present such as hunger, discomfort, perhaps pain, and transient or permanent impaired function caused by conditions or treatment. Therefore the window for interplay may be limited by the physical and psychological energy of the infant to engage.

I always proceed with caution in providing new experiences for a newborn in the hospital. Where an infant shows interest such as turning towards the therapist, transient or fixed eye contact, or becoming still, I may make the transition into singing. The transition is cautiously achieved by increasing the melodic nature of a spoken phrase into a semi-sung motif (Shoemark and Grocke 2010). This may include a wider range of pitches, lengthened durations on any one pitch, or increasing the sense of tonal structure by centring the speech around a tonic. If the infant continues to show interest, I may introduce a single sung melodic line (Shoemark 2008). Likewise, the tempo, rhythm, pitch and timbre of the melody emulate the tempo, rhythm, pitch and timbre of the spoken phrase. In both instances, there will also be silence, a pause, to allow for a lagged response from the infant, before deciding whether to transition into singing or maintain the interplay where it is. The lyrics will basically retain the words of the spoken phrase to minimize the novel stimuli.

The following story is taken from a description of a session with Andrew, an infant aged 8 weeks old (Shoemark 2008). It was our eleventh session and we had previously experienced a good level of attunement. This example illustrates the moment just before infant-directed speech becomes infant-directed singing.

Andrew had endured a period of several minutes in which he was quite upset. He had protested well and begun to withdraw from the interplay, but I had managed to gently keep him in the interplay in the hope that I could soothe his escalating distress and calm him perhaps towards sleep:

Helen feels that Andrew has not got the organizational energy to cope with interaction now. She thinks helping him to make a transition to sleep or a Quiet Alert state may be the best option. 'Time for sleeping' Helen states [to him], with a nod of her head and a pause. 'Is that the story?' she asks, then pauses. Andrew keeps his eyes firmly on Helen, but lightly moves his fingers on Helen's hand. She responds in kind with her fingers while keeping eye contact with him.

Helen transforms the spoken phrase into a slower and more rhythmic chant 'A <u>time</u> for <u>sleep</u>-ing a-<u>gain</u> . . . I think.' It is a recitative like phrase, accompanied by rhythmically matched bottom patting. Andrew calmly watches Helen, entranced by the chant. So Helen consolidates its role by repeating it. His breathing finally settles. Now she knows they are on the right path. She continues to pat his bottom in time and smile as she makes her voice more breathy, and slows the chant down.

'Yeah?' she asks, as if waiting for Andrew to tell her he was ready to sleep. She adjusts the location of her left hand to make her little finger available to his right hand. He immediately takes hold of her little finger and watches her. As Helen repeats the chant one more time the words are more pitched and it finally becomes melodic. Here is the shifting point into lullaby.

The interaction is intimate in its moment-by-moment development. However as therapist, most steps are anticipated and constructed, rather than spontaneously occurring. The therapist can rapidly process the interplay to determine the present factors and to take the next step to attain the objective of the moment. The subtlety of music and musicality is ideally suited to this attention to minute details of interplay.

Without the unpleasant tasks of nursing care to perform, and without the emotional roller coaster of parental attachment to endure, the music therapist is uniquely placed to provide both a consistently positive self and a consistent range of positive interaction. The therapeutic dyad comes together in the shared experience of speech and singing which quickly becomes predictable and familiar and serves as an intrinsically safe place which requires no further conscious processing of the experience on the part of the infant, but affords opportunity to be and change through just 'doing' (Morgan 1998). As Morgan suggests '(f)rom a dynamic systems approach, it is the small changes the bring about the large changes' (Morgan 1998 p. 330).

Conclusion

Pavlicevic noted that a mother and infant 'need to share meaning: to have a common experience of themselves and one another, so that the infant may experience itself within the context of the relationship' (1997 p.101). In the NNU the starting point for every infant is a critical medical status which requires significant medical intervention. There is little prospect of the mother and infant sharing quality experiences as many infants are ventilated and/or sedated. We are yet to completely understand what impact this early, but perhaps only brief experience has on the mother–infant dyad's experience of each other as articulated by Pavlicevic. Potentially, the neonatal music therapy service creates the opportunity to reconnect mother and infant employing the otherwise naturally occurring patterns of interpersonal communication as a simple guide to protect them both in their efforts towards contingency. As the attuned relationship and companionship makes little demand on the infant, the presence of the music therapist as an additional relationship in the infant's life aims to provide a sustaining force for the infant's sense of self and well-being.

References

Abrams, B., Dassler, A., Lee, S., Loewy, J., Silverman, F., and Telsey, A. (2000). Instituting music therapy in NICU: a team centred approach. In J. Loewy (ed.) *Music Therapy in the Neonatal Intensive Care Unit*, pp. 21–38. (New York: Satchnote)

Ainsworth, M.D.S., Blehar, M.C., Waters, E., and Wall, S. (1978). *Patterns of Attachment: a Study of the Strange Situation*. (Hillsdale, NJ: Erlbaum)

Als, H. (1996). *Program Guide—Newborn Individualized Developmental Care and Assessment Program (NIDCAP): an Education and Training Program for Health Care Professionals*. (Available from National NIDCAP Training Center, Harvard Medical School, Children's Hospital, Boston, MA, USA)

Beebe, B. and Lachmann, F. (1994). Representations and internalizations on infancy: three principles of salience. *Psychoanalytic Psychology*, 11, 127–165.

Beebe, B., Jaffe, J., Lachmann, F., Feldstein, S., Crown, C., and Jasnow, M. (2000). Systems models in development and psychoanalysis: the case of vocal rhythm coordination and attachment. *Infant Mental Health Journal*, 21, 99–122.

Beebe, B., Knoblauch, S., Rustin, J., and Sorter, D. (2005). *Forms of Intersubjectivity in Infant Research and Adult Treatment*. (New York: Other Press)

Blumenfeld, H., and Eisenfeld, L. (2006). Does a mother singing to her premature baby affect feeding in the Neonatal Intensive Care Unit? *Clinical Pediatrics*, 45, 65–70.

Bowlby, J. (1969). *Attachment and Loss: Volume 1: Attachment*. (London: Hogarth)

Crown, C., Feldstein, S., Jasnow, M., Beebe, B., and Jaffe, J. (2002). The cross-modal co-ordination of interpersonal timing: six-week-olds infants' gaze with adults' vocal behavior. *Journal of Psycholinguistic Research*, 31, 1–23.

De Casper, A., and Fifer, W. (1980). Of human bonding: newborns prefer their mothers' voices. *Science*, 208, 1174–1176.

de l'Etoile, S. (2006). Infant behavioral responses to infant-directed singing and other maternal interactions. *Infant Behavior & Development*, 29, 456–470.

Fegran, L., Helseth, S. and Solveig Fagermoen, M. (2008). A comparison of mothers' and fathers' experiences of the attachment process in a neonatal intensive care unit. *Journal of Clinical Nursing*, 17, 810–816.

Fernald, A. (1989). Intonation and communicative intent in mothers' speech to infants: is the melody the message? *Child Development*, 60, 1497–1510.

Fernald, A., and Kuhl, P. (1987). Acoustic determinants of infant preference for motherese speech. *Infant Behavior & Development*, 10, 279–293.

Fifer, W., and Moon, C. (1994). The role of mother's voice in the organization of brain function in the newborn. *Acta Paediatrica*, 397, 86–93.

Griffin, T. (2006). Family-centered care in the NICU. *Journal of Perinatal and Neonatal Nursing*, 20, 98–102.

Hall, E. (2005). Being in an alien world: Danish parents' lived experiences when a newborn or small child is critically ill. *Scandinavian Journal of Caring Sciences*, 19, 179–185.

Harris, J. (2005). Critically ill babies in hospital–considering the experience of mothers. *Infant Observation*, 8, 247–258.

Hepper, P., and Shahidullah, B. (1994). Development of fetal hearing. *Archives of Disease in Childhood*, 71, F81–F87.

Hurst, I. (2001). Mothers' strategies to meet their needs in the newborn intensive care nursery. *Journal of Perinatal and Neonatal Nursing*, 15, 65–83.

Jaffe, J., Beebe, B., Feldstein, S., Crown, C., and Jasnow, M. (2001). Rhythms of dialogue in infancy: co-ordinated timing in development. *Monographs of the Society for Research in Child Development*, 66, 1–132.

Kaminski, J., and Hall, W. (1996). The effect of soothing music on neonatal behavioral states in the hospital newborn nursery. *Neonatal Network*, 15, 45–54.

Lillas, C. and Turnbull, J. (2009). *Infant/Child Mental Health, Early Intervention, and Relationship-Based Therapies*. (New York: W.W. Norton & Co.)

Longhi, E. (2009). 'Songese': maternal structuring of musical interactions with infants. *Psychology of Music*, 37, 195–213.

Malloch, S., Shoemark, H., Newnham, C., Črnčec, R. Paul, C., Prior, M., Coward, S., and Burnham, D. (in press). Music therapy with hospitalised infants–the Art and Science of Intersubjectivity. *Infant Mental Health Journal*.

McGrath, J. (2001). Building relationships with families in the NICU: exploring the guarded alliance. *Journal of Perinatal and Neonatal Nursing*, 15, 74–84.

Miles, M., Holditch Davis, D., Burchinal, P., and Nelson, D. (1999). Distress and growth outcomes in mothers of medically fragile infants. *Nursing Research*, 48, 129–140.

Moon, C., and Fifer, W. (2000). Evidence of transnatal auditory learning. *Journal of Perinatology*, 20, 37–44.

Morgan, A. (1998). Moving along to things left undone. *Infant Mental Health Journal*, 19, 324–332.

Nakata, T., and Trehub, S. (2004). Infants' responsiveness to maternal speech and singing. *Infant Behavior and Development*, 27, 455–464.

Ockleford, E., Vince, M., Layton, C., and Reader, M. (1988). Responses of neonates to parents' and others' voices. *Early Human Development*, 18, 27–36.

O'Gorman, S. (2007). Infant-directed singing in neonatal and paediatric intensive care. *Australia and New Zealand Journal of Family Therapy*, 28, 100–108.

Papoušek, H., and Papoušek, M. (1991). The meanings of melodies in motherese in tone and stress languages. *Infant Behavior and Development*, 14, 415–440.

Parker, S., Zahr, L., Cole, J., and Brecht, M. (1992). Outcome after developmental intervention in the NICU for mothers of preterm infants with low socioeconomic status. *Journal of Pediatrics*, 120, 780–785.

Pavlicevic, M. (1997). *Music Therapy in Context: Music, Meaning and Relationship.* (London: Jessica Kingsley)

Rock, A., Trainor, L., and Addison, T. (1999). Distinctive messages in infant-directed lullabies and play songs. *Developmental Psychology*, 35, 527–534.

Rose, H., and Mayer, J. (1968). Activity, caloric intake, fat storage and the energy balance of infants. *Pediatrics*, 41, 18–29.

Sameroff, A., and Fiese, B. (2000). Transactional regulation: the developmental ecology of early intervention. In S.J. Miesels, and J.P. Shonkoff (eds) *Handbook of Early Childhood Intervention*, pp. 135–159. (Cambridge: Cambridge University Press)

Sameroff, A., Bartko, W., Baldwin, A., Baldwin, C., and Seifer, R. (1998). Family and social influences on the development of child competence. *Psychoanalytic Dialogues*, 5, 579–593.

Schore, A. (1994). *Affect Regulation and the Origin of the Self: the Neurobiology of Emotional Development.* (Hillsdale, NJ: Erlbaum)

Seideman, R., Watson, M., Corff, K., Odle, P., Haase, J., and Bowerman, J. (1997). Parent stress and coping in NICU and PICU. *Journal of Pediatric Nursing*, 12, 169–177.

Shoemark, H. (2006). Infant-directed singing as a vehicle for regulation rehearsal in the medically fragile full-term infant. *Australian Journal of Music Therapy*, 17, 54–63.

Shoemark, H. (2008). Mapping progress within an individual music therapy session with full-term hospitalized infants. *Music Therapy Perspectives*, 26, 39–46.

Shoemark, H., and Dearn, T. (2008). Keeping the family at the centre of family-centred music therapy with hospitalised infants. *Australian Journal of Music Therapy*, 19, 3–24.

Shoemark, H. and Grocke, D. (2010). The markers of interplay between the music therapist and the medically fragile newborn infant. *Journal of Music Therapy*, 47, 306–334.

Spence, M., and Freeman, M. (1996). Newborn infants prefer the maternal low-pass filtered voice, but not the maternal whispered voice. *Infant Behavior & Development*, 19, 199–212.

Stern, D. (1985). *The Interpersonal World of the Infant.* (New York: Basic Books)

Stern, D., Spieker, S., and MacKain, K. (1982). Intonation contours as signals in maternal speech to prelinguistic infants. *Developmental Psychology*, 18, 727–735.

Stewart, K. (2001). A Transpersonal Approach to Music Therapy in the Neonatal Intensive Care Unit. Unpublished thesis, New York University, New York.

The Royal Children's Hospital Melbourne (2010). About the RCH Neonatal Unit. Available at http://www.rch.org.au/neonatal_rch/index.cfm?doc_id=6933Inpatient_Clinical_Services. Accessed 3 May 2010.

Trainor, L., Clark, E., Huntley, A., and Adams, B. (1997). The acoustic basis of preferences for infant-directed singing. *Infant Behavior & Development*, 20, 383–396.

Trainor, L., Austin, C., and Desjardins, R. (2000). Is infant-directed speech prosody a result of the vocal expression of emotion? *Psychological Science*, 11(3), 188–195.

Trehub, S., and Schellenberg, E. (1995). Music: its relevance to infants. *Annals of Child Development*, 11, 1–24.

Trehub, S., Unyk, A., and Trainor, L. (1993a). Adults identify infant-directed music across cultures. *Infant Behavior & Development*, 16, 193–211.

Trehub, S., Unyk, A., and Trainor, L. (1993b). Maternal singing in cross-cultural perspective. *Infant Behavior & Development*, 16, 285–295.

Trehub, S., Unyk, A., Kamenetsky, S., Hill, D., Trainor, L., Henderson, J., and Saraza, M. (1997). Mothers' and fathers' singing to infants. *Developmental Psychology*, 33, 500–507.

Trevarthen, C. (2001). Intrinsic motives for companionship in understanding: their origin, development and significance for infant mental health. *Infant Mental Health Journal*, 22, 95–131.

Tronick, E. (1998). Dyadically expanded states of consciousness and the process of therapeutic change. *Infant Mental Health Journal*, 19, 290–299.

Winnicott, D.W. (1964). *The Child the Family and the Outside World*. (Harmondsworth: Penguin)

Chapter 12

Music therapy for hospitalized infants and their parents

Joanne V. Loewy

Daniel's birth at 33 weeks was sudden and unexpected. Tasha had been in the park with her friends and at approximately 2.30 a.m. she felt severe 'pain and flutters' and noticed vaginal bleeding. With assistance from her friends, Tasha limped to the Emergency Room of the hospital and had an emergency delivery. Although Tasha denied drug use, urine toxicology indicated that Tasha had used methadone with frequency within the past 2 months. At the time of Daniel's music therapy assessment, Tasha, still hospitalized, was on 24-h watch on the maternity unit, and was scheduled to be transferred to the psychiatric unit because she had reportedly declared to staff that she intended to kill herself. Tasha had reported to the resident doctor that she had used drugs in high school but had been 'clean' for the past 5 years.

Introduction

Human beings begin the course of existence tuning in to another human being. In the first moments of development, we synchronize our patterns of growth in accordance with the womb environment where we exist referentially, adapting to the rhythms of another. Experiences in the womb, at birth and during early childhood profoundly affect the long term physical, emotional and mental health of human beings (Penman 1983; Francis and Meaney 1999; Weinstock 2005; Hernández-Martínez et al. 2008). Brain and nervous system development, immune system fortitude, as well as cognition and learning capacity including the development of coping strategies, emotional stability and physical coordination are critically interdependent (Schore 1994; Porges 1998, 2002).

Traumatic circumstances can interrupt growth and development. Infants of pregnant mothers who absorb physical and emotional stress are often born with predisposing vulnerabilities (Porges 1998). This also applies in the case of drug using parents whose infants are born addicted, resulting in the diagnosis of neonatal abstinence syndrome (NAS). Research supports the impact of emotional factors such as loss, fear, and/or depression which impede healthy growth and development (Insel and Young 2001).

The influence of mood and the regulation of physical health practices are becoming a routine part of prenatal care. As anxiety and unresolved conflicts during pregnancy may have negative effects on the progress of labour and the incidence of obstetric complications, McKinney (1990) and also Hanser and colleagues (Hanser et al. 1983), provided some of the earliest reports of the relevance of music therapy during pregnancy. McKinney (1990) provided a review of music therapy for women during pregnancy citing three studies: Guided Imagery and Music (GIM) (Linquist 1985); music therapy using directed imagery and recorded music (Winslow 1986); and progressive muscle relaxation using recorded music (Liebman 1989). This review provided insight about how music therapy was used in prenatal care at this time of the history of the development of music therapy practices (McKinney 1990).

Infants and parents who experience risk may be faced with traumatic challenges. This is especially true for premature babies where the necessity for medical interventions often requires that they be separated from their parents (Stewart 2010). In these circumstances, parents are at high risk for developing depression (Hernández-Martínez et al. 2008). The inability to bond can result from this physical separation impeding the natural course of development for both baby and parent. This may, in turn, interfere with the beginning stages of healthy emotional growth.

Attachment: the neurobiology of deprivation and abuse in child development

Research in many countries has validated the importance of healthy attachment between parent and child (Bowlby 1982; Coleman and Watson 2000). Music therapy can provide an important means for achieving stability by offering a natural incentive for attaining and securing healthy attachments which provide a basis for the development of trusting relationships (Stern et al. 1982; Ribaupierre 2004).

Aside from medically influenced circumstances which may present unavoidable risks for vulnerable premature babies and young children, traumatic instances of poor attachment also can result from a parent not being present, or the presence of an unhealthy familial attachment. This typically is experienced in the form of deprivation, neglect or abuse. Though case reports in the literature may reflect that neglect is highest amongst families of lower economic status, neglect can also exist in higher income status families where the primary caregivers are unavailable, or where narcissistic tendencies pervade the environment (Luthar and Lattendresse 2005). In such instances basic nurturing practices may be absent. Recurring passive avoidance profoundly affects the young child's brain capacity to develop normally resulting in psychopathology (Carter and Keverne 2002).

Trauma

Early relational trauma can also be caused by active abuse, such as sexual abuse, physical assault, or emotional abuse. Schore (2003) is a psychobiologist who has outlined how fear and terror resulting from such interpersonal trauma results in the development of a destructive core belief system about oneself and others. This may lead to an inability to create and experience safe and meaningful attachments. A lack of attachment may include symptoms such as limited empathy resulting in a poor sense of shared experience, or an inability to bond (Schore 2003). Schore described the arrest of attachment and regulation as leading towards an inability to manage conflict. This could result in the tendency to be fearful of relationships in adult life, and might bring forth a sense that interpersonal relations are either 'insubstantial, suffocating, or simply impossible to obtain' (Schore 2003 p. 133).

The strong emerging neurobiological theoretical basis which recognizes potential vulnerability in early development has been welcomed in music therapy. Porges, a neurobiologist who has specialized in trauma research has defined the importance of the amygdala, the part of the brain responsible for timing the information that travels to the cortex (Porges 2008). Overloading the amygdala with information can cause chronic stress responses and can be destructive to the memory function of the hippocampus. The trauma-inducing events that have occurred are not 'time tagged' and can be re-experienced instantly when a trigger is encountered.

The role of the right prefrontal cortex is essential in the development of positive relationships, as is the dorsolateral frontal cortex. The Polyvagal Theory (Porges 2001) offers an explicit neurobiological model of how 'difficulties in spontaneous social behavior are linked to both facial expressivity and the regulation of visceral state, and alternatively, how social behavior may serve as a regulator of physiological activity' (Porges 2001 p. 36). Behaviour and physiology are linked. Therefore physical reactions can stimulate parent–infant interactions that are important for the infant's learning about how to self-regulate.

Polyvagal theory proposes that the evolution of the nervous system determines not only the range of one's emotional experience but also the quality of communication and the ability to regulate bodily and behavioural states (Porges 2001). This contributes to the theoretical justification for the role that music therapy can play in activating neural circuits that regulate reactivity. Porges' rationale for and description of feeding and rocking as primal attachment behaviours which influence vagal afferent pathways is an essential contributor to the current thinking about the importance of the quality of care in the first stage of life. Music therapy practices that activate somatomotor components which trigger visceral change influence attachment practices which are critically important in the early years. Porges describes rocking's importance in providing an 'efficient and direct influence on the vagas by stimulating vagal afferent pathways via baroreceptors' (Porges 2001 p. 35).

Music therapy in the neonatal intensive care unit (NICU): the roots of attachment

The foetus is part of a system, dependent upon the physiological condition of another human being. Considering this from both medical and music therapy perspectives working within the meter of respiratory and cardiac rates of both mother and foetus in the context of an entrainment model has important synchronous medical implications (Loewy 2004).

The life rhythm of the heart beat is the first sound that a developing foetus hears in the womb. The significance of a steady pulse has been noted as a primary means of awareness, as in the concept of basic beat (Nordoff and Robbins 2007), involving high level neurological processing (Grahn and Brett 2007). Rhythm can affect movement in older adults (Tomaino 2000; de l'Etoile 2010), and can assist in speech for people who have dementia (Clair 1996). The influence of rhythm is indicated and mapped in the brain and is thought to influence organization which is helpful in studying cognition and brain plasticity (Münte et al. 2002; Grahn and Brett 2007).

Complementary medicine programmes have incorporated aspects of rhythm and breath work into specific methods to enhance relaxation in pregnant women (Hanser et al. 1983). Breath attunement has been effectively influenced through music therapy (Loewy 2005). Since the body actively uses respiratory mechanisms to play wind instruments and to sing or tone, the use of these applications can be monitored and physiologically served through music therapy when the foetus is in the womb, as well as when the infant is outside the mother's body. Purposeful sustenance of the musical aspects of this environment can provide continuity thus sustaining the rhythmic, flowing components.

At Beth Israel Medical Center, music therapy was established in the NICU in 1999. *Heather on Earth* clinical trials have combined two tracks of intervention; medical music therapy and music psychotherapy. The medical music therapy interventions include implementation of live music entrained to the premature infant's heart rate and respiratory rate. The Remo ocean disc and gato box have been part of the sound environment that our music therapists have incorporated in accordance with the recommendations of the team comprised of the neonatologists, nurses, social workers, nutritionists, and physical therapists (Loewy 2000). Interventions are made according to diagnosis, and care is clustered within day-to-day treatments. The music therapy team has included parents and caregivers as often as possible in the development of entrained lullabies which are sought to be culturally specific to the familial song of kin (Loewy et al. 2006, 2009).

One of the most essential music psychotherapy strategies in the NICU is the music therapist's work with parents. In most circumstances, the therapist meets with parents and will assess their level of stress. A crucial aspect of this evaluation is to understand how aspects of the unknown such as fear, separation and/or a lack of power or frustration might influence the parents' level of stress. So many parents of premature infants experience worry or fear. This is often accompanied by a sense of loss, and/or control which is at times further confounded by an unconscious sense of shame or blame related to the birth circumstances of their infants.

Understanding the unique aspects of each parent's crisis which led to premature delivery is essential to a music therapist's capacity to intervene with the parent and baby in a meaningful way. Furthermore, knowing what melodies are preferred and working with parents to show them how to tone, and most sensitively intervene, can be a wonderfully therapeutic means of empowerment between therapist and parent. This parallel process provides useful skills in transferring these gentle interventions to their babies. Additionally, the music therapist may learn the timbre and melodic range of mother and father's speaking and singing voice. Recording the parents' voices can be helpful in providing a tonal and timbral range of familiarity which can be easily employed by the therapist. As the parents' confidence in these musical interactions builds, the music therapist can assist them in creating a recording of favourite lullabies for use several times a day in the incubator. This may serve especially useful in circumstances in which parents cannot be present for session work with their infants.

Infants who are born to mothers who are chemically dependent often present as critically ill. Additionally, they may be physically addicted to the agents ingested *in utero*. Infants born with NAS typically present a host of difficult needs medically, physiologically, and emotionally. Irritability and nervous system agitation require special attention. In cocaine use, the infant may be under-reactive, sleeping more than the average infant. In methadone use, infants might have trouble sleeping, and high-pitched crying for long periods is not unusual. These infants often require neonatal opium solution (NOS) or phenobarbital in order to manage their symptoms and gradually withdraw from the dependency.

Poor attachment behaviours between the mother and infant impacts later learning. Difficulties in the ongoing child's growth and development are often observed. Attachment may be critically threatened for these babies as they may be removed early in life from the care of their parent(s) by the Association for Child Services (ACS).

Case study—Daniel: NAS, respiratory distress syndrome (RDS), gestational age 33 weeks, corrected age 3 weeks

Daniel's birth at 33 weeks was sudden and unexpected. Tasha had been in the park with her friends and at approximately 2.30 a.m. she felt severe 'pain and flutters' and noticed vaginal bleeding. With assistance from her friends, Tasha limped to the Emergency Room of the hospital and had an emergency delivery. Although Tasha denied drug use, urine toxicology indicated that Tasha had used methadone with frequency within the past 2 months. At the time of Daniel's music therapy assessment, Tasha, still hospitalized, was on 24-h watch on the maternity unit, and was scheduled to be transferred to the psychiatric unit because she had reportedly declared to staff that she intended to kill herself. Tasha had reported to the resident doctor that she had used drugs in high school but had been 'clean' for the past 5 years.

Daniel was born to a 21-year-old, Tasha, who had two younger children. Tasha lived with her mother and husband along with her two older sisters in the lower east side of Manhattan. Daniel's father, Chad, aged 23, had worked as a cashier in a supermarket in Brooklyn, but returned to Trinidad, his native country 8 months prior to Daniel's birth. Tasha had received her GED (graduate equivalency degree) at age 19. She had spent recent years raising her 4-year-old son and 2-year-old daughter. Tasha's mother was supportive of her daughter but had a heart attack 4 months prior to Tasha's delivery of Daniel. At the time of Daniel's birth, Tasha's mother was home but on bed rest with complications of diabetes and reportedly with a 'fragile heart'. Daniel was referred to music therapy because he was reportedly irritated; screaming 'round the clock' according to one nurse. The social worker had concerns that Daniel had had no visitors and indicated that the mother was still on ACS hold.

At the time I set out to first work with Daniel, I found him in the infant swing. The nurses indicated that being in the swing was 'the only thing that would stop his crying' for short periods. As I observed Daniel, and reviewed his medical record, I listened to the pitch and tone of his screaming, and began to think of past referrals of NAS. How often these infants benefit from stimulating sound, and frequent and direct interventions. Based on my past experiences on this ward, Daniel seemed to need motion and tone, entrained to the timbre and pitch, a perfect 5th below his cry.

This is a common need for infants who are born dependent on pharmacologic agents. Music therapy can provide stimulatory experiences within a holding environment. Before performing an assessment with baby Daniel, I asked the social worker where I could find his mother Tasha, and she referred me to the maternity unit, as Tasha had not as of yet been transferred to the psychiatric unit. My intention in meeting Daniel's mother was to hear the tonality and range of her voice, and also learn about any music that Daniel may have been exposed to during pregnancy. I also wanted to seek any songs or lullabies of importance to her; melodies and experiences that she had found meaningful with her other children.

Music therapy with Tasha

Tasha eagerly accepted me and music therapy into her room. Although her bag was packed as she awaited transfer, the mere offer of music therapy, and the sight of my cart of musical instruments brought up what seemed to be tears of relief and thanks: 'I just cannot see Daniel like this—or my others . . .' I assured her that I had come to play for her. After a grounding warm up, we discussed the music that I might bring to Daniel, until she gained her strength back. I noticed her voice was mezzo-soprano (mid-c to g) range and had a nasal lyrical quality.

She said her musical love was Bob Marley's 'Stir it Up.' She spoke of her mother, who according to Tasha, had been recently moved to her great aunt's, and she mentioned her worry related to her other children who were with their aunt. Her biggest fear was an awareness that she might not have Daniel with her when she eventually left the hospital. 'I cannot see my new baby like this . . . I am, a mess'. When our discussion had reached the point where the details of Tasha's fears were being repeated and seemingly perpetuating more fear, I asked her to simply assist me in developing a lullaby for Daniel: 'How would that be?' I asked. 'Just great . . .' she replied, releasing a deep breath.

I asked her to sing 'Stir it Up' as she liked it to be sung. 'I cannot sing—trust me' was her first reply. In the key of where she had spoken this (G), I began to strum in reggae style on the guitar and playfully sang back to her: 'you say you can't sing, but we're gonna try . . .'.

I sang this several times in G and then segued to A and started improvising with the lyrics of her chosen song, 'stir it up . . . little darling', 'stir it up . . . oh yeah, dear Tasha, how shall we, stir on up . . . dear dear Tasha, it's been a long long time, since we had you on our mind, oh yeah . . .'.

Tasha smiled and began singing. She sang back the words and we were playful and improvisatory for many verses which related to having Daniel on her mind. She sang about her other children. Eventually, she accepted my offer to focus on creating a lullaby that I would use specifically with Daniel, until the point where she would feel ready to visit her son in the NICU. Using the sedation effect (Loewy 2009) and demonstrating how 'Stir it Up' could be simplified into a 6/8 holding meter, and the lyrics with melody brought into two lines: 'Stir it up . . . little Daniel, stir it up . . . Danny boy . . .' Tasha and I sustained these lyrics and simple melody into the lullaby I would later use to soothe him.

By the time transport came to wheel her to the psychiatric unit, Tasha had assurances that I would be singing her lullaby to Daniel, and I also offered to return to her, in the psychiatric unit, to make a recording of her singing the lullaby. I assured her that we could place it in Daniel's bassinet and that he would hear her familiar voice. She was grateful.

There are multiple ways that the music therapist can guide live music therapy sessions with parents such as demonstrating how breath tones on the sound 'aah' can assist their baby's breathing process, or showing how the meter of their breathing patterns can influence their infant's breathing. These techniques can be helpful for parents in building attunement and strength. In the case of Daniel, who had respiratory distress in addition to NAS, the 'aah' and perhaps ocean disc would be significant to try. I was also most interested in providing 'Stir it Up' in A as it had been developed with his mother. I saw my role and the role of music therapy as a transitional object (Winnicott 1953).

Music therapy with Daniel

Daniel was crying when I entered his room. His cry tones were uneven. The nurse said he had not been holding down his feed which is common for premature infants as the digestive tract is immature. I watched and listened to the accents of his cry and the pulsed urgent meter of his tones. I determined it as a fussy cry.

I first began by simply singing on 'aah' and carefully observed his reaction. I used this tone again with the ocean disc, attuning my tone to his cry, in an expanded tonal vocal hold (Loewy 1995) with Daniel. After three of these 'aah's, he turned his head toward me and I sensed that he wanted to be held as his left foot bent slightly up into his belly. Putting down the ocean disc, I lifted him and cradled him into my arms and we toned for a while before moving into the lullaby. Daniel's need for nurturance was apparent. As his eyes gazed into mine, I pictured Tashsa's face and tone and sang: 'Stir it up . . . little Daniel', etc. Daniel's lullaby was soothing and we rocked slightly. I thought of how this movement had supported him, and the difference between the swing and my arms and vibrating tones. After 30 min or so, Daniel's eyes began to look heavy. I entrained the lullaby to match his breathing and following the sedation effect (Loewy 2005), toned out with the word 'Danny' as he fell off to sleep. The following week, Tasha and I created a lullaby tape, which I assured her would be used by the team with Daniel several times a day.

Summary

Tasha eventually began supervised visits with her son, and she was discharged. Her diagnosis of depression and enrolment in a rehabilitation programme on an outpatient basis was mandated by the ACS, especially as the care of her other children in her present state was being questioned. Daniel was not discharged to his home as the authorities found his mother to be 'unfit': that is, a risk to his safety. There was a possibility he would be put up for adoption in future months. Such cases are the reality of working in an inner city where social support for patients is minimal.

Promoting relationships to enhance attachment and bonding, only then to witness abrupt separations between newborns and parents can be difficult in music therapy practice. Yet, the earliest moments of life and the potential of music to provide essential roots of stimulatory significance strengthens a human being's capacity to grow. The strength of music in providing nurturance between mother and baby is never a wasted therapeutic effort, even when separation may be an eventual inevitable outcome. Musical nurturance is durable and can transmit safety amidst such traumatic separations.

The importance of music therapy in the bonding process is critical for the development of the child. In the earliest moments of life, the impact of music can be life affirming. This case reflects music therapy interventions that serve both medical (RDS, ocean–womb live sounds entrained), and emotional (mother impetus, live lullaby with attachment impact) aspects of care.

Music therapy NICU interventions

The Remo ocean disc was described briefly above. In general, the ocean disc is meant to replicate the whooshing sounds of the uterus. Since parents do not have this instrument readily available at home, music therapy sessions can demonstrate for parents how their own breath sounds, provided on 'ah' can be equally nurturing, particularly for infants who are having difficulty breathing.

Additionally, the gato box can provide a rhythm tapped lightly to the infant's breathing or heart rate. This can be soothing for both infants and parents as their systems are physiologically and emotionally comingled via natural entrainment (Rider 1997). Demonstrating the comfort of a steady meter and showing how a gentle rhythmic light pat on their infant's back while holding the infant over the heart can be part of the demonstrations and instructions given to parents. For mothers who are in hospital, comfort and relaxation are often compromised. Lack of sleep might exacerbate tension and cause physical and emotional complications. Using mechanisms of meter as a context for entraining, music can be used in a variety of ways to assist fragile parents in their ability to provide a relaxed, nurturing sound environment which can assist in their achieving a deep sleep state for their baby (Courtnage et al. 2002).

Providing nurturance through favourite lullabies designed for parents is critical at this time. Initiating a point of contact using a lullaby is highly personal. Beginning from playing in a familiar meter and moving into a holding meter, and then to a rubato style, music's ability to contain, and gradually withhold the need for a fixed predictable meter can assist in the creation of a relaxation effect, which can be achieved in a very short period of time (Loewy 2009).

Interweaving music medicine and music therapy interventions within a music psychotherapy approach is an integrative way of practising. Combining knowledge of diagnoses and adherence to vital signs when providing live ocean and womb sounds (active entraining), yet instituting an individually based treatment that caters to the cultural and specific music preferences is critical.

Conclusion

Music medicine and music psychotherapy approaches provide a myriad of unique opportunities for infants and children especially as they are treated within a family-centred care context. Integral to our treatment is the understanding we can provide through careful assessment and evaluation of the infants' means of attachment and in the safety we can seek to establish in the honouring of developing bonds. This honouring is easily fulfilled in notation and sound, but the psychotherapeutic aspects of its institution require observation, knowledge of infant/child development (which is inclusive of knowledge of musical skill development), as well as an understanding of trauma and how significant issues may present with opportunity for resolution in musical play. This chapter has provided an integration of music psychotherapy intervention in a context where the development of attachment is best realized through analyses of both parent and child. In this way we can seek to build and strengthen theory and application of how the body's natural use of music can play a conscious and realized role in the unfolding relationship between parent and child.

References

Bowlby, J. (1982). *Attachment and Loss*, 2nd Edn. (New York: Basic Books)

Carter C.S., and Keverne E.B. (2002). The neurobiology of social affiliation and pair bonding. In D. Pfaff (ed.) *Hormones, Brain and Behavior*, pp. 299–337. (San Diego: Academic Press)

Clair, A. (1996). Effect of singing on alert responses in persons with late stage dementia. *Journal of Music Therapy*, 33, 234–247.

Coleman P., and Watson, A. (2000). A Reply to Commentaries on 'Infant attachment as a dynamic system'. *Human Development*, 43, 327–331.

Courtnage, A., Chawla, H., Loewy, J.V., and Nolan, P. (2002). Effects of live infant directed singing on oxygen saturation, heart rate, and respiratory rate of infants in the neonatal intensive care unit. Abstract 2346. *Pediatric Research*, 51, 403A.

de l'Etoile, S.K. (2010). Neurologic Music Therapy: a scientific paradigm for clinical practice. *Music and Medicine*, 2, 78–84.

Francis, D., and Meaney, M. (1999). Maternal care and the development of stress responses. *Current Opinion in Neurobiology*, 9, 128–134.

Grahn, J., and Brett, M. (2007). Rhythm and beat perception in motor areas of the brain. *Journal of Cognitive Neuroscience*, 19, 893–906.

Hanser, S., Larson, S., and O'Connell, A. (1983). The effect of music on relaxation of expectant mothers during labor. *Journal of Music Therapy*, 20, 50–58.

Hernández-Martínez, C., Arija, V., Balaguer, A., Cavallé, P., and Canals, J. (2008). Do the emotional states of pregnant women affect neonatal behaviour? *Early Human Development*, 84, 745–750.

Insel, T.R., and Young, L.J. (2001). The neurobiology of attachment. *Nature Reviews Neuroscience*, 2, 129–136.

Liebman, S. (1989). The effects of music and relaxation on third trimester anxiety in adolescent pregnancy. Unpublished doctoral thesis, Miami, FL.

Linquist, R. (1985). The role of GIM in the birthing process. Unpublished fellows paper, Institute for Music and Consciousness, Townsend, WA.

Loewy, J.V. (1995). The musical stages of speech: a developmental model of pre-verbal sound making. *Music Therapy*, 13, 47–73.

Loewy, J.V. (2000). *Music Therapy in the NICU.* (New York: Satchnote Armstrong Press)

Loewy, J.V. (2004). A clinical model of music therapy in the NICU. In M. Nocker-Ribaupierre (ed.) *Music Therapy for Premature and Newborn Infants*, pp. 159–176, trans. S. Weber. (Gilsum, NH: Barcelona)

Loewy, J.V. (2009). Musical sedation: mechanisms of breathing entrainment. In R. Azoulay, and J.V. Loewy (eds) *Music, the Breath & Health: Advances in Integrative Music Therapy*, pp. 223–232. (New York: Satchnote Press)

Loewy, J.V., Hallan, C., Friedman, E., and Martinez, C. (2005). Sleep/sedation in children undergoing EEG testing: a comparison of chloral hydrate and music therapy. *Journal of PeriAnesthesia Nursing*, 20, 323–332.

Loewy, J.V., Hallan, C., Friedman, E., and Martinez, C. (2006). Sleep/sedation in children undergoing EEG testing: a comparison of chloral hydrate and music therapy. *American Journal of Electroneurodiagnostic Technology*, 46, 343–355.

Luthar, L., and Latendresse, S. (2005). Children of the affluent: challenges to well-being. *Current Directions in Psychological Science*, 14, 49–53.

McKinney, C. (1990). Music therapy in obstetrics: a review. *Music Therapy Perspectives*, 8, 57–60.

Münte, T.F., Altenmüller, E., and Jäncke, L. (2002). The musician's brain as a model for neuroplasticity. *Nature Neuroscience Reviews*, 3, 473–478.

Nordoff, P., and Robbins, C. (2007). *Creative Music Therapy: A Guide to Fostering Clinical Musicianship.* (Gilsum, NH: Barcelona)

Penman, R., (1983). Synchronicity in mother-infant interaction: a possible neurophysiological base. *British Journal of Medical Psychology*, 56, 1–7.

Porges, S. (2002). Dysregulation of the right brain: a fundamental mechanism of traumatic attachment and the psychopathogenesis of posttraumatic stress disorder. *Australian and New Zealand Journal of Psychiatry*, 36, 9–30.

Porges, S. (2008). The polyvagal theory: new insights into adaptive reactions of the autonomic nervous system. *Cleveland Clinic Journal of Medicine*, 75, 81–85.

Porges, S.W. (1998). Love: an emergent property of the mammalian autonomic nervous system. *Psychoneuroendocrinology*, 23, 837–861.

Porges, S.W. (2001). The polyvagal theory: phylogenetic substrates of a social nervous system. *International Journal of Psychophysiology*, 42, 123–146.

Ribaupierre, M.N. (2004). *Music Therapy for Premature and Newborn Infants.* (Gilsum, N.H.: Barcelona)

Rider, M. (1997). Entrainment music, healing imagery, and the rhythmic language of health and disease. In J. Loewy (ed.) *Music Therapy in Pediatric Pain*, pp. 81–88. (Cherry Hill, NJ: Jeffrey Books)

Schore, A. (1994). *Affect Regulation and the Origin of the Self: The Neurobiology of Emotional Development.* (Mahwah, NJ: Lawrence Erlbaum)

Schore, A. (2003). *Affect Dysregulation and Disorders of the Self.* (New York: W.W. Norton)

Stern, D., Speiker, S., and MacKain, K. (1982). Intonation contours as signals in maternal speech to prelinguistic infants. *Developmental Psychology*, 18, 727–735.

Stewart, K. (2010). Music therapy, the preterm infant and the spectrum of traumatic experiences. In K. Stewart (ed.). *Music Therapy and Trauma: Bridging Theory and Clinical Practice*, pp. 131–151. (New York: Satchnote Armstrong Press)

Tomaino, C. (2000). Working with images and recollection with elderly patients. In D. Aldridge (ed.) *Music Therapy in Dementia*, pp. 195–211. (London: Jessica Kingsley)

Weinstock, M. (2005).The potential influence of maternal stress hormones on development and mental health of the offspring. *Brain Behavior and Immunity*, 19, 296–308.

Winnicott, D.W. (1953). Transitional objects and transitional phenomena. A study of the first not-me possession. *International Journal of Psycho-Analysis*, 34, 89–97.

Winslow, G. (1986). Music therapy in the treatment of anxiety in hospitalized high-risk mothers. *Music Therapy Perspectives*, 3, 29–33.

Chapter 13

Music therapy supports parent–infant attachments: In families affected by life threatening cancer

Clare O'Callaghan and Brigid Jordan

. . . when parents with cancer are hospitalized they may borrow instruments to play with their infants during their visits, altering otherwise potentially boring visiting times for the children and enabling shared family fun. Parents can be given charts with letters for their infants' favourite songs, such as 'Twinkle, Twinkle'. Parents can learn to play these tunes on instruments like the metallaphone for their child during their visits. This conveys to the infant that the parent is thinking of them even though they are separated by hospitalization, which is important to promote 'good enough' attachment experiences.

Introduction

The inattention to support for parent–child interactions in hospice literature and related clinical work has been described as 'woeful' (Saldinger et al. 2004). The situation in oncology is comparable, especially in regard to the needs of infants and toddlers, aged 4 years and younger. The burden of children of parents with life threatening illnesses is potentially greatest, as they are dependent on their parents for their physical and emotional well-being (Saldinger et al. 2004); more poignantly so during infancy.

An infant's cancer treatment experience and potential death can also be devastating and exhausting for parents, as families strive to get through each day, with grief and hope juxtaposed, or one emotion supplanting the other, as the illness ameliorates or progresses. Medical advances have prolonged the time that many people live until they die, and families and patients may prepare themselves for death, but then the patient unexpectedly recovers. The uncertainty and extended anticipatory grief can be harrowing for all, whatever the eventual outcome (Boog and Tester 2008).

Locating the lens: music therapy practice contexts

Music therapy can be defined as the creative and professionally informed use of music in a therapeutic relationship with people identified as needing physical, psychosocial, or spiritual help, or with people aspiring to experience further self-awareness, enabling increased life satisfaction and quality (O'Callaghan in press). The first author has worked since 1985 as a music therapist in two cancer treatment, and three palliative care settings—one of which was a home-based service. These contexts have included adult and paediatric cancer treatment services, as well as adult inpatient hospices, and an all ages home-based palliative care service. Her work has been characterized by part-time jobs with large client bases, and ongoing self-reflection about the most useful way that her particular skills and time could be spent.

In these hospice and cancer care settings music therapy needs to be flexibly available, as patients' conditions fluctuate and, especially in inpatient oncology, there can be unexpected interruptions to patients' schedules, including unexpected tests, treatments, visitors, and discharges. Music therapy is therefore often characterized by endeavouring to 'catch the therapeutic possibilities' as one can. In these settings referrals are made by staff or patients and members of their families (O'Callaghan 2006). Inpatient sessions may be held at patients' bedsides and in chemotherapy day wards. The consequent potential intrusive effects of open ward sessions need to be monitored, especially when young visitors are involved, although in the first author's experience neighbouring patients usually welcome the 'life affirming' presence of children.

Infants with cancer

From 1997 to 2006 in Australia, almost half of the children under 15 years of age who were diagnosed with cancer were in infancy; with 223 infants per million diagnosed during that period (Cancer Council Queensland). As parents and children are interdependent, the experience of one influences the other. Child characteristics, various coping factors such as family cohesion and social supports (Klassen et al. 2007), and optimistic outlook (Maurice-Stam et al. 2008) are related to parental health when caring for children up to 18 years old with (Klassen et al. 2007) or in remission from cancer (Maurice-Stam et al. 2008). There is scant attention, however, to the particular vulnerabilities endured by infants with cancer and their families, although it is known that pre-existing family factors are important to the adjustment of all involved (Kazak and Baxt 2007). Some parents have indicated a sense of relief that their children are young and hope that they will not remember the treatment (Kazak and Baxt 2007). The clinical experience of the authors shows that infants can find it more difficult, compared with older children, to understand what has happened to their bodies, the need for hospitalization and treatments, and the reasons for restriction of activities. Parents may express concern that their children might not be able to describe their symptoms. Additionally parents can find it difficult to administer treatments as needed.

Infant survivors of cancer, their parents, and many siblings are vulnerable to post-traumatic stress symptoms (PTSS), which can include re-experiencing traumatic memories of the child's illness and treatment. Kazak and Baxt (2007) have suggested a three-phase model of intervention to reduce or prevent PTSS. In the first phase, during the initial stage of cancer diagnosis, interventions are directed at reducing exposure to associated traumatic elements, for example promoting effective pain management, and supporting the family's coping resources. In phase two, interventions are directed at identifying children and families at risk for continuing PTSS and alleviating their distress. In phase three, after the conclusion of the initial cancer treatment, the goal is to address the ongoing distress and support positive adaptation (Kazak and Baxt 2007).

Mothers of infants with life limiting conditions can be especially vulnerable to trauma and distress. Mothers can experience the conflict of loving and becoming securely attached to the child while knowing and imagining expected separation, and this ambivalence and mourning state can compromise the mother's capacity to contain, hold, and reassure the child. Fathers may act protectively to the mother and infant and may feel helpless or even a failure when the mother is distressed and the baby is terminally ill. Some parents attempt to cope by doing physical tasks rather than directly engage with the baby (Boog and Tester 2008). Infants under 2 years old cannot conceptualize the permanency of death, and this may remain difficult in the 2- to 5-year-old age group, with the young child expecting the dead person to return (Raphael 1984).

To promote infant mental health and healthy future development, infant–parent psychotherapy approaches have advanced from only focusing on the parent without directly engaging the infant, to regarding the baby as independent in his or her own right. Working with the parent and child together facilitates a healthy relationship between them; it promotes 'a space which enables growth' (Thomson-Salo and Paul 2004 p. 27). When an infant is psychologically vulnerable, therapeutic work is regarded as urgent. This is because the longer the negative experiences remain unmodified, the more likely there will be adverse and enduring neural effects (Perry et al. 1995). When so much energy goes into keeping the infant alive during cancer treatment, opportunities for 'normal' playful exchanges between parents and infants are reduced, further exposing the infant to vulnerability in being able to develop a securely attached relationship with their parents.

Prolonged infant separation from primary caregivers, especially when the infant is very unwell and enduring painful medical procedures, is also a traumatic experience that, unaddressed, can increase the risk of adverse neurodevelopmental outcomes, including persisting hyperarousal and/or dissociative symptoms (Perry et al. 1995). Children's reactions to separation are noted as even more intense when they are in pain (Magill et al. 1997). It is imperative that supportive care modalities address the misunderstanding that 'children are resilient' (Perry et al. 1995) and enable their best possible adaptation:

> Children are not resilient, children are malleable. In the process of 'getting over it' elements of their true emotional, behavioural, cognitive, and social potential are diminished—some percentage of capacity is lost, a piece of the child is lost forever (Perry et al. p. 285).

Infant mental health therapists work with strategies that promote healthy parent–infant interaction, including the power of using gaze and play. Thoughtfully looking at the infant in an attempt to understand something of their experience will often enable the infant to feel that they have received something of value that supports their development of an awareness of 'self' and 'other' (Thomson-Salo et al. 2004 p. 16). Similarly, when an infant–parent dyad is 'stuck', or unable to fully engage, it may indicate that the child's sense of playfulness is vulnerable, and that if the therapist brings a sense of fun, play, and creativity to the child, the child's own playfulness can be restarted, also igniting the parent and infant's shared play (Thomson-Salo and Paul 2004). As Winnicott (1971) has noted, it is only through playing that the child is able to be creative and discover the self.

Parents with cancer

Parents living with cancer have described profound impacts on their lives, including worries about uncertain futures, fear of death, stressors associated with role changes and fatigue (Helseth and Ulfsaet 2005; Elmberger et al. 2008), and the conflicting demands of being a good parent and patient. Mothers have described their interpretations of their children's fears, including fear about their hospitalizations (Elmberger et al. 2008), while fathers in one study did not tend to notice their children's reactions (Elmberger et al. 2002). Parents coping with cancer diagnosis and treatment often try to protect their children and try to help them to feel secure and normal, leading to a recommendation that strategies need to be developed that help patients feel like good parents (Helseth and Ulfsaet 2005). There has been little focus in the literature to date on how to help parent–child communication when the parent has cancer at any age (Turner et al. 2007), and parents can experience difficulty knowing how much information to give their children about what is happening (Elmberger et al. 2000). A brochure with suggested communication strategies, notably the recommendation to 'tell them that you love them', was developed in Queensland, Australia, following in-depth interviews with parents with advanced cancer (Turner et al. 2007).

When it is the case that cancer enters the final stage, parents and their children can yearn for close connection. Final farewells can be an important means of helping the 'survivors-to-be' maintain healthy attachments to their parent following their death. However, research indicates that family coping can sometimes be associated with denial of the impending death rendering it difficult for professionals to facilitate family connectedness through this time (Saldinger et al. 2004). The parent and child need to be psychologically able to face nearing death in order to share time together for successful 'anticipatory relationship facilitation'; that is, supporting the child's continuing attachment with their parent after the death (Saldinger et al. 2004).

Swick et al. (2006) found that helping the parents with end stage cancer to find the language to communicate with their children can facilitate their children's adjustment. Parents are encouraged to create legacies for infants (Swick et al. 2006; Boog and Tester 2008). As infants will construct a significant part of their view of the deceased parent based on others, it is also important to identify adults who will be available on an ongoing basis to help them know who their parent was (Swick et al. 2006).

Attachment

The major emotional and social tasks through infancy include learning to regulate emotions and to form close and secure attachment relationships. Reliable emotional availability and sensitive and responsive caregiving by parents promotes the infant's sense of security and provides the foundation for emotional health (Ainsworth 1985). Parents with cancer may struggle to remain consistently emotionally available and responsive to their infant due to the emotional demands of and preoccupation with the emotional impacts of their grave illness. Infant reactions to caregiver absences and distress, and disruptions in routines, can result in eating and sleeping problems, tearfulness, tantrums, especially at separation times such as bedtimes, regression to earlier developmental changes (Swick and Rauch 2006), and clingy behaviours (Boog and Tester 2008). Threats to the development of a secure attachment relationship between infant and parent include precipitous and extended separations beyond the developmental capacity of the infant to cope (Bowlby 1969). Although infants do not have an understanding of death, the nature of the attachment relationship between parents and infants, and the infant's experience of separation and loss can reverberate throughout the child's future life. Infants who experience traumatic separation and loss may have emotional disturbances that continue into adult life (Bowlby 1988; Boog and Tester 2008). Neurobiological responses to trauma may in turn affect their emotional and social functioning (Perry et al. 1995). Therefore, it is incumbent on health professionals to assist in the development of healthy and enduring family connectedness and relationships where possible (Boog and Tester 2008). Health professionals should support: (a) parents being able to mitigate the adverse consequences of their ill health and separation on their children's mental health, in the immediate and long-term future; and (b) the needs of infants with cancer being responded to, including their distress not being intensified by the parents' uncontained emotions.

Grief and bereavement

Grief comprises the painful personal feelings and suffering associated with loss, while bereavement is the loss of the relationship, and includes overall adaptation to the loss (Christ 2000; Boog and Tester 2008). Earlier theories, grounded in the work of Freud, Bowlby, and Parkes declared that mourning and adjustment to loss was characterized by moving forward and detachment, that is, 'letting go of the relationship that can no longer be sustained in life' (Boog and Tester 2008 p. 74). Such detachment has been relabelled as 'reorganization' in recent writings, or a 'relocation of the deceased' person, enabling adjustment to their physical absence in ongoing life. One should not leave the deceased behind, but reintegrate the lost relationship into one's present internal world and life (Stroebe and Schut 1999 p. 198).

Coping with loss involves a dynamic process of grieving, a waxing and waning that includes yearning and 'taking time off from grieving' (Stroebe and Schut 1999 p. 212), and 'restoration-orientation', which includes the mastery of tasks related to adjustment (Stroebe and Schut 1999).

This model indicates that there is no set bereavement pattern for anyone. Anticipatory grief, that is, grieving before the mortal loss, may also occur, potentially affecting parents' attachment to their critically ill infants in distressing ways, and infants may display behavioural and emotional disturbances when distressed by this inconsistency in parental availability.

Music therapy supporting parent–infant attachments affected by cancer

The literature review presented here indicates that music therapists involved with infants and parents, when either is affected by cancer, should aim to support their connectedness and relationship. There are time frames therapists may consider when aiming to do this, including: (a) in 'here-and-now' moments when working with the parent and child; (b) when working individually with the child or parent to create a music therapy 'product', which can later be shared with their loved one(s), so as to convey the message that they are in each other's minds; and (c) when working individually with the parent to create a legacy. This legacy of story or song and/or poetry can communicate to the infant their parent's recognition of the importance of the infant to the parent, the significance of this relationship for both infant and parent, and how the parent may be integrated into their infant's life in the future, should the parent die.

Music therapy with infants who have cancer

Boog and Tester (2008) have urged that 'every effort should be made to create a soft, comfortable and nurturing environment' (p. 35) for the parents to be with their infants who are seriously ill, including a comfortable chair, soft lighting, baby items, and gentle music. This may include the necessity for a staff member to be available for parents who need additional support. Music therapists may have helpful suggestions for the types of music that parents could play with their child, and also enquire about the music that the parents may have attachments to from their own childhood, that nurtured them, and which can potentially sustain them now.

Some parents may prefer unfamiliar music to support and validate their availability at this time, and appreciate being offered varying music genres. Therapists also need to be aware that infants with brain involvement may be sensitive to some music and frequencies which can trigger seizures (Sweeney-Brown 2005). Sweeney-Brown (2005) has illustrated how music therapists can profoundly support parent–infant attachment through helping the parent share live music with their infant. Catherine provided music therapy to James, who was blind as a result of a tumour which formed when he was 9 months old. Towards the end of his life, at the age of 4, James was irritable and in severe pain but relaxed and slept for short periods when the parents held him while Catherine sang or played the flute. When reflecting about these experiences Catherine later wrote, 'His family still refer to these sessions as positive memories in the midst of a difficult time' (p. 54). One can only imagine the support that these session memories offered James' parents as they potentially remembered doing all they could to be available for James and comfort his distress. Catherine also described how she sometimes held James.

Music therapists may also model music attachment behaviours for parents (O'Callaghan et al. in press) which can be helpful when distressing health circumstances thwart parents' 'aliveness' with their infant, and the baby is not very responsive to them. When parents witness engagement between the therapist and baby, the parents see that there is hope and may make sufficient internal shifts to be able to respond to the baby's need (Thomson-Salo and Paul 2004).

Dun's (2007) description of how she created a music therapy space, enabling a mother to contain, reassure, and support her 5-year-old daughter awaiting bone marrow transplantation, provides important insights into how music therapy can support parent–infant attachments in paediatric oncology.

> She was huddled into her mother . . . whimpering . . . . I sang songs that are well-known to 5 year olds, keeping my guitar accompaniment simple . . . and my voice gentle . . . . As I sang, the mother began to rock Olivia gently back and forth . . . Eventually Olivia looked out from her safe haven to check me out and when she did this I gently engaged Olivia with some duck castanets which she played herself, appearing less anxious, smiling and sitting upright on her mother's lap. Her mother was also smiling and interacting with Olivia. (Dun 2007)

Olivia's story exemplifies Dun's description of her effectiveness as a music therapist through being a 'bricoleur', that is one who 'joins children (and arguably parents) on their journeys . . . (being) in the moment with them meeting their immediate and emerging needs, while holding them as a person . . . throughout that journey and creating possibilities.' (Dun 2007).

The first author's (Clare) previous work with children attending radiotherapy treatment and their families is also one where the music therapy methods were adapted to the needs and desires of those who chose to be involved (O'Callaghan et al. 2007). These children often came to the waiting area while preparing and having radiotherapy treatment for 6 weeks, and for follow-up treatments. Instruments were scattered around the waiting area and Clare would tend to wait to see whether the infant approached the instruments with or without their parents. If parents and infants played together, Clare would affirm and possibly offer assistance to support their musical shared process. For example, when the child grew bored with one instrument, Clare would offer another instrumental sound, or she would teach the parent how to help their child activate the movement sensitive musical sounds (and noises) on a keyboard, which often elicited guffaws of laughter in both parents and their children. Some parents 'plonked' in the comfortable arm chairs and watched Clare improvise music or share songs with their children, and Clare would look for opportunities to offer the parents support. This may have been through engaging their child in music therapy while they rested and 'quietly' read a magazine, or the parents may have described issues related to the cancer experience, which sometimes led to referrals to other multidisciplinary team members. Through supporting the parent, one is supporting the infant, as their potential to be available to meet their child's needs may be strengthened.

Sometimes parents found new ways of musically relating to their children in these sessions, and asked where to buy the instruments they played. Family song making usually included the child's suggestions of lyrics, although parents and siblings would also sometimes add their thoughts.

Sometimes this needed delicate negotiation as Clare tried to support all people being 'heard'. As Aasgaard (2005) has described in his work with children with malignant blood diseases, some songs are created in the moment together without being put down in writing, and a helpful and 'safe' way to get started is through lyric substitution; where new lyrics are created for an existing song. Clare often invited older infants and toddlers, and sometimes their families, to start song writing with a simple melody that was an exaggeration of the natural inflexions of the child's speaking voice, with I, IV, and V accompanying chords, 4/4 time. A standard lyrical framework often used when engaging young patients was:

> Today a met a girl/boy called . . .
> Who loves to . . .
> And . . .
> And . . .
> And s/he has a dad/mum/friend/dog called . . .
> Who loves to . . .

Children were offered multiple choice or closed-ended questions to elicit answers which were then included in the lyrics. Sometimes a bridge would be created that was easy for everyone to sing, for example, animal sounds of their pets, or audible expressions of favourite activities described. Sometimes these songs were recorded with the children singing, for which parents were grateful. Sometimes this song writing would also inspire more original songs. Many of the songs, while potentially described as 'play songs' or even 'nonsense songs', actually described family relationships. The recording would often be played in the car on journeys home from hospital, offering further opportunities for the infant and parent to share precious time in normal and fun interactions. The song recordings could offer delight to the parent who was unable to attend the hospital, for example because of work responsibilities, presumably because they now could hear how they were held in their child's mind. This can reinforce their value at a time when parents can feel helpless, as the cancer trajectory feels so much out of their control.

Occasionally the songs became legacies as some children sadly died. These songs may then offer some consolation for the bereaved. Memories of such happy times in music therapy sessions may also comfort bereaved parents (Lindenfelser et al. 2008).

Parents with cancer

Magill described groundbreaking music therapy work in partnership with a social work colleague that enabled hospitalized parents with cancer to connect with and respond to their distressed and isolated infants, supporting both the infants and their families. One of the case studies included a 3-year-old boy, Michael, who, having not seen his dying hospitalized mother for 3 months, developed a stutter, became aggressive in play, highly dependent on other adults, and regularly searched the house for 'mommy'. The immediate need to bring the family together was identified after the mother went into a semi-comatose state. The social worker prepared the infant and his 6-year-old sibling to visit their mother with their father and, after they entered her room, Magill arrived and sang family requested songs, conveying the message, 'I hear you'. The music especially calmed the atmosphere when the children sang together with their father as they sat by and touched their mother. The children's special messages to their mother and each other were conveyed through word lyric substitution in songs, such as 'He's Got the Whole World in his Hands', and their mother 'responded to their touch and the sound of the music by blinking her eye that had filled with tears.' (p. 35). The children continued these visits for 2 weeks until their mother died, the father became more attentive to their needs, the children expressed their concerns and fears more openly, and Michael stuttered less and his play was less agitated (Slivka and Magill 1986).

Music therapy and social work clearly played an integral role in supporting Michael and his sibling's grief experience. Through responding to their fears and concerns, alongside creating a therapeutic space for mother–child connectedness, the children felt acknowledged, known, and loved. The children could know that the mother's separation from them was not her wish, that she would be with them if it was not for the cruelty of fate, and this knowing, according to attachment theory, will help them to reorganize their relationship with their mother in their bereavement as one who, while no longer there, loved them, and would be with them if she could be.

Two decades after Michael's story was published, fewer parents die in acute treatment cancer hospitals, as many are discharged to palliative care programmes, but they seldom have much energy in either setting, due to treatment side effects or advancing disease. In oncology and palliative care work, Clare looks for opportunities to assist parent–infant connectedness, and much can be accomplished in 'one-off sessions'.

Adult cancer outpatients have also attended the radiotherapy waiting area open-ended music therapy sessions, described earlier, and shared musical improvisation and play, and song writing in comparative ways with their infants. Sharing familiar play songs, including actions, can also inspire parent–infant interactions. The music therapist endeavours to create a music space to help support that interaction, but may share the primary connection with the healthy infant when the parent needs a break. This may include spending time with infants in the waiting areas while the parents have consultations with their medical specialists.

> Julie noted that her two infant sons (4 and 2 years old) hated coming to Peter Mac, Australia's only sole cancer treatment and research centre, while she came for her 6 weekly check-ups for symptom management related to a melanoma diagnosis. After meeting the music therapist, Pip Barry, she could leave her children in the waiting room so that she could have a private discussion with her doctor, while the children happily engaged in fun, creative free play with a range of musical instruments with Pip. When Julie returned to the waiting area, she also musically interacted with her sons and Pip, and sometimes reflected on her cancer experiences, whereupon Pip would offer support. Julie reported that the sessions helped her to get the children ready to come to Peter Mac as they looked forward to their music therapy sessions.
>
> (Pip Barry, personal communication, 13 May 2008)

Parents may also benefit from observing the infant's 'aliveness' when interacting with a playful music therapist especially if the parents are struggling to recapture their own sense of fun and play with their infant. Parents may appreciate the music therapist helping them to initiate their own musical improvisation and song sharing with their infants. While a music therapist may feel concerned that the parent could feel worse watching the music therapist playfully interact with their infant, if the parents felt that that they were not having comparable times with them, the infant mental literature suggests that parents can, in fact, feel relieved when they observe such connectedness, and are encouraged to initiate similar experiences with their infants in the future (Thomson-Salo and Paul 2004).The music therapist may also provide CDs and instruments which can facilitate the parent–child's interaction and connectedness outside the music therapy session.

Song writing is a way for parents separated from infants to convey important messages. Song writing allows parents to state what they want their children to know, in a way that is tolerable to the parent (O'Callaghan et al. 2009), which is vitally important when one considers that denial is a form of coping with the devastating experience of dying and leaving young children (Saldinger et al. 2004). For example, one woman, who was close to dying, wrote a series of songs for her young children. She described many of her memories with them, expressed compliments, described her love for them, and advised them about who they could turn to in the future. However, she was not 'ready' to tell them her hopes for their futures.

Through song writing, parents may metaphorically communicate messages in developmentally appropriate ways. In some music therapy sessions parents have composed songs telling their infants that they will remain available in the stars after their deaths (O'Brien 2003; O'Callaghan et al. 2009). These songs may also become lullabies, as they are offered to children to help them sleep.

Inviting parents to write lyrics to the tune of 'Twinkle, Twinkle, Little Star' may enable the song writing process, especially if a parent identifies that this song is one of their child's favourites.

When the parent is separated by hospitalization, the song compositions can be given to the spouse, or another carer, for them to use with the child, to remind the child of the separated parent, potentially helping them to sleep, as the song becomes a lullaby, and eventually perhaps, a soothing lament (O'Callaghan 2008). Alternately, parents may write songs for use when their child gets older, with adult themes and messages (O'Callaghan et al. 2009).

A secure attachment history is associated with successfully negotiating developmental life tasks and, arguably, these songs can help the children in their development should the parent die, because they know their parents loved them and would continue to be with them if it was not for the fickleness and cruelness of fate. In a number of the songs written by parents for the infants (and older children) parents describe their memories and beliefs that they will remain with them in some form. This may help to consolidate one's memory of feeling known by the parent. As Winnicott (1971) has proposed, when a child feels known, they can feel fully alive and may more successfully creatively adapt to being in the world. Swift (2006) has stated that one of the most important things for bereft infants to know is who is available for them. In some of their parents' song compositions, the parents express the memory of being available and the wish to be available, and who their children can turn to for support (O'Callaghan et al. 2009).

There are a range of approaches described for helping parents to write songs for their children (O'Callaghan 1996; Dileo and Magill 2005; O'Brien 2005), and to help children receiving treatment for cancer to write songs (Aasgaard 2005). Little attention in song writing, however, has focused on which person should record the songs. Clare encourages parents to record the songs for their children but sometimes they are reluctant, deriding their singing voices. In some cases the parents will sing, but this may require support. One parent, for example, was more welcoming of the recording of her song when her voice and accompanying drumming was accompanied by Clare's singing.

Melodies that exaggerate the parent's natural speaking voice inflections may also help. The audible sounds, and images and feelings conveyed in the lyrics, can accompany the infant in their journey and, should the parent die, be reworked over time to support life stage transitions. Parents are often delighted by hearing their thoughts and feelings being transformed into songs for their children. They are often surprised and proud of the product, and pleased that their messages are in songs. Parents, including surviving spouses, may wonder when the 'right' time might be for their children to hear the songs. They can be reassured that the songs are for when the time 'feels right' which may not be for a long time, if ever.

Discussion

Cancer health professionals need to consider creative ways that parental and infant distress may be alleviated when cancer affects their lives. Music therapists who work with songs, improvisation, and song writing with children, elicit important information useful for psychosocial assessments within a multidisciplinary team. Music therapy experiences described in this chapter demonstrate that many of the therapeutic strategies recommended for parent–infant attachments under duress can be provided, including the use of music for reigniting shared play, and normal shared fun and interactions (Thomson-Salo and Paul 2004), and musical messages of love (Turner et al. 2007). Parents can feel good about themselves through successfully writing songs (Helseth and Ulfsaet 2005). Music therapy methods may also be used to educate older infants about treatment experiences, regarded as important to prevent PTSS (Kazak and Baxt 2007), and descriptions of cancer treatments can be integrated into songs.

Despite Saldinger's (2004) suggestion that professionals can find it difficult to promote 'anticipatory relationship facilitation' between parents with advanced illnesses and their infants, it is evident that music therapists can enable a 'language' (Swick and Rauch 2006) that can allow many of these dyads to hear, feel, and know that they are in each other's minds, directly or indirectly, in psychologically tolerable ways. Song writing can also include messages about who the infant can turn to which may support the developing child's internalization of an emotionally available parent figure, associated with healthy life task negotiation (Winnicott 1971; Grossmann 1999; Swick and Rauch 2006). Case examples like those described here can be used to justify funding for music therapy as a supportive care modality in the poorly addressed area of parent–infant well-being in oncology. Varying theoretical perspectives indicate that music therapy supported interactions can favourably affect the current and future mental health of parents and infants enduring cancer treatment.

Addressing supportive care needs of infants experiencing attachment difficulties in an oncology context reduces the potential to develop the emotional and neural impacts that are associated with poorer long-term mental health. When these care needs are identified and addressed at an early enough stage mental health vulnerability can be reduced (Perry et al. 1995), ultimately potentiating a healthier and happier future.

Further research to better understand music therapists' potential role in supporting healthy parent–infant attachments in oncology could include (a) lyric analyses of songs conjointly written by the parents and infants, (b) textual analysis of interviews of parent song writers' experiences creating these songs, and (c) infants' experiences of their parents' songs in years to come. Case study analyses of infants involved in music therapy sessions with hospitalized parents, or who receive songs from them, may also offer interesting insights. For example, exploring the experience of an adult bereaved at 18 months of age who has kept the song his father wrote with the lyrics, 'My greatest legacy is you, thank you for making my life whole and complete'. It may also be important to discover the experience of parents who have music therapy legacies created by their infants. What is it like for parents to have a recording with their deceased 4-year-old daughter singing about a joyful birthday party they gave her?

There is scant information about later effects of infancy cancer survival, however it is speculated that these effects will be burdensome (Barr 2007), notably as the young age is a risk factor for more severe late effects including physical, neurocognitive, and associated emotional and social effects (Perry et al. 1995; Kazak and Baxt 2007). The responsiveness of infants to musical interactions would indicate that appropriate psychosocial and psychotherapeutic interventions can alter their situation positively (Perry et al. 1995; Thomson-Salo and Paul 2004), and address any potential parent–infant attachment problems. The development of effective interventions for better therapeutic outcomes for young cancer survivors is recommended (Barr 2007).

Music therapy methods, including therapeutic music lessons, song writing, improvisation, and familiar songs, make important contributions in this area. In particular, music therapy may promote positive neural, cognitive, emotional, and social development (O'Callaghan et al. 2007) and could be considered an essential part of any infant cancer survivor's rehabilitation and psychological recovery.

Conclusion

One of the most profoundly distressing aspects for parents with life threatening cancer is imagining that they will not be around to see their children grow up. Parents with infants with life threatening conditions may be so consumed by their own distress, fear, and anticipatory grief that they find it difficult to respond to the comfort needs of their children. Music therapy offers a range of methods that support parent–infant connectedness and attachment; promoting healthy relating and providing comfort for the work of adjustment which follows.

Music therapy can help parents and infants who are affected by life threatening cancer. Music therapy allows the experience of helpful musical moments, strategies, and legacies. This enables parents and infants to live more adaptively in the time available together and if ultimately separated, this prior experience can support infants' negotiation of future developmental transitions while easing the experience of bereavement.

References

Aasgaard, T. (2005). Assisting children with malignant blood disease to create and perform their own songs. In F. Baker and T. Wigram (eds) *Songwriting: Methods, Techniques and Clinical Applications for Music Therapy Clinicians, Educators and Students*, pp. 154–179. (London: Jessica Kingsley)

Ainsworth, M.D.S. (1985). Patterns of infant-mother attachments: antecedents and effects on development. *Bulletin of New York Academy of Medicine*, 61, 771–791.

Barr, R.D. (2007). Editorial. Difficult beginnings - cancer in infancy. *Pediatric Blood & Cancer*, 49, 1059.

Boog, K.M., and Tester, C.Y. (2008). *Palliative Care: a Practical Guide for the Health Professional*. (Edinburgh: Churchill Livingstone)

Bowlby, J. (1969). *Attachment and Loss: Volume 1: Attachment*. (London: Hogarth Press)

Bowlby, J. (1988). Developmental psychiatry comes of age. *American Journal of Psychiatry*, 145, 1–10.

Cancer Council Queensland. A summary of childhood cancer incidence in Australia 1983–2006. Available at http://www.cancerqld.org.au/icms_docs/60378_A_Summary_of_Childhood_Cancer_Incidence_in_A ustralia_1983–2006.pdf. Accessed 11 May 2010.

Christ, G.H. (2000). *Healing Children's Grief: Surviving a Parent's Death from Cancer*. (New York: OUP)

Dileo, C., and Magill, L. (2005). Songwriting with oncology and hospice adult patients from a multicultural perspective. In F. Baker and T. Wigram (eds) *Songwriting: Methods and Clinical Applications for Music Therapy Clinicians, Educators and Students*, pp. 226–245. (London: Jessica Kingsley)

Dun, B.J. (2007). Journeying with Olivia: bricolage as a framework for understanding music therapy in paediatric oncology. *Voices: a World Forum for Music Therapy* Available at http://www.voices.no/mainissues/mi40007000229.php. Accessed 30 April 2008.

Elmberger, E., Bolund, C., and Lutzen, K. (2000). Transforming the exhausting to energizing process of being a good parent in the face of cancer. *Health Care for Women International*, 21, 485–499.

Elmberger, E., Bolund, C., and Lutzen, K. (2002). Men with cancer: changes in attempts to master the self-image as a man and as a parent. *Cancer Nursing*, 25, 477–485.

Elmberger, E., Bolund, C., Magnusson, A., Lutzen, K., and Andershed, B. (2008). Being a mother with cancer: achieving a sense of balance in the transition process. *Cancer Nursing*, 31, 58–66.

Grossmann, K.E. (1999). Old and new internal working models of attachment: the organization of feelings and language. *Attachment and Human Development*, 1, 253–269.

Helseth, S., and Ulfsaet, N. (2005). Parenting experiences during cancer. *Journal of Advanced Nursing*, 52, 38–46.

Kazak, A., and Baxt, C. (2007). Families of infants and young children with cancer: a post-traumatic stress framework. *Pediatric Blood & Cancer*, 49, 1109–1113.

Klassen, A., Raina, P., Reineking, S., Dix, D., Pritchard, S., and O'Donnell, M. (2007). Developing a literature base to understand the caregiving experience of parents of children with cancer: a systematic review of factors related to parental health and well-being. *Support Care Cancer*, 15, 807–818.

Lindenfelser, K., Grocke, D., and McFerran, K. (2008). Bereaved parents' experiences of music therapy with their terminally ill child. *Journal of Music Therapy*, 45, 330–348.

Magill, L., Coyle, N., Handzo, G., and Loscalzo, M. (1997). Cancer and pain: a creative multidisciplinary approach in working with patients and families. In J. Loewy (ed.) *Music Therapy and Pediatric Pain*, pp. 107–114. (Cherry Hill, NJ: Jeffrey Books)

Maurice-Stam, H., Oort, F.J., Last, B.F., and Grootenhuis, M.A. (2008). Emotional functioning of parents of children with cancer: the first five years of continuous remission after the end of treatment. *Psycho-Oncology*, 17, 448–459.

O'Brien, E. (2003). *Living Soul* (CD). (Melbourne: Crystal Mastering)

O'Brien, E. (2005). Songwriting with adult patients in oncology and clinical haematology. In F. Baker and T. Wigram (eds) *Songwriting Methods, Techniques and Clinical Applications for Music Therapy Clinicians, Educators and Students*, pp. 185–205. (London: Jessica Kingsley)

O'Callaghan, C. (1996). Lyrical themes in songs written by palliative care patients. *Journal of Music Therapy*, 33, 74–92.

O'Callaghan, C. (2006). Clinical issues: music therapy in an adult cancer inpatient treatment setting. *Journal of the Society for Integrative Oncology*, 4, 57–61.

O'Callaghan, C. (2008). Lullament: lullaby and lament therapeutic qualities actualized through music therapy. *American Journal of Hospice & Palliative Medicine*, 25, 93–99.

O'Callaghan, C. (2010). The contribution of music therapy to palliative medicine. In G. Hanks, N. Cherny, N. Christakis, M. Fallon, S. Kaasa, and R. Portenoy. (eds) *The Oxford Textbook of Palliative Medicine*, 4th Edn, pp. 214–221. (Oxford: Oxford University Press)

O'Callaghan, C., Sexton, M., and Wheeler, G. (2007). Music therapy as a non-pharmacologic anxiolytic for paediatric radiotherapy patients. *Australasian Radiology*, 51, 159–162.

O'Callaghan, C., O'Brien, E., Magill, L., and Ballinger, E. (2009). Resounding attachment: cancer inpatients' song lyrics for their children in music therapy. *Support Care Cancer*, 17, 1149–1157.

O'Callaghan, C., Baron, A., Barry, P., and Dun, B. (in press). Music's relevance for pediatric cancer patients: a constructivist and mosaic research approach. *Support Care Cancer*. doi: 10.1007/s00520-010-0879-9.

Perry, B.D., Pollard, R.A., Blakley, T.L., and Vigilante, D. (1995). Childhood trauma, the neurobiology of adaptation, and 'use-dependent' development of the brain: how 'states' become 'traits'. *Infant Mental Health Journal*, 16, 271–291.

Raphael, B. (1984). *The Anatomy of Bereavement: a Handbook for the Caring Professions.* (London: Hutchinson and Co.)

Saldinger, A., Cain, A., Porterfield, K., and Lohnes, K. (2004). Facilitating attachment between school-aged children and a dying parent. *Death Studies*, 28, 915–940.

Slivka, H.H., and Magill, L. (1986). The cojoint use of social work and music therapy with children of cancer patients. *Music Therapy*, 6, 30–40.

Stroebe, M., and Schut, H. (1999). The dual process model of coping with bereavement: rationale and description. *Death Studies*, 23, 197–224.

Sweeney-Brown, C. (2005). The beginnings of music therapy in our hospice. In M. Pavlicevic (ed.) *Music Therapy in Children's Hospices: Jessie's Fund in Action*, pp. 48–61. (London: Jessica Kingsley)

Swick, S., and Rauch, P. (2006). Children facing the death of a parent: the experiences of a parent guidance program at the Massachusetts General Hospital Cancer Center. *Child and Adolescent Psychiatric Clinics of North America*, 15, 779–794.

Thomson-Salo, F., and Paul, C. (2004). Some principles of infant-parent psychotherapy: Ann Morgan's contribution. In F. Thomson-Salo and C. Paul (eds) *The Baby as Subject: New Directions in Infant-Parent Psychotherapy from the Royal Children's Hospital, Melbourne*, pp. 27–40. (Melbourne: Stonnington Press)

Thomson-Salo, F., Paul, C., Morgan, A., Jones, S., Jordan, B., Meehan, M., Morse, S., and Walker, A. (2004). 'Free to be playful': therapeutic work with infants. In F. Thomson-Salo and C. Paul (eds) *The Baby as Subject: New Directions in Infant-Parent Psychotherapy from the Royal Children's Hospital, Melbourne*, pp. 9–26. (Melbourne: Stonnington Press)

Turner, J., Yates, P., Hargraves, M., and Hausmann, S. (2007). Development of a resource for parents with advanced cancer: what do parents want? *Palliative and Supportive Care*, 5, 135–145.

Winnicott, D.W. (1971). *Playing and Reality.* (London: Routledge).

Index